Innovation in Action

A practical guide for healthcare teams

Innovation in Action

A practical guide for healthcare teams

D. Scott Endsley, MD, MSc

Director, Innovation and System Design
Cleveland Clinic
Cleveland, Ohio
USA

WILEY-BLACKWELL

A John Wiley & Sons, Ltd., Publication

BMJ|Books

This edition first published 2010, © 2010 by D. Scott Endsley

BMJ Books is an imprint of BMJ Publishing Group Limited, used under licence by Blackwell Publishing which was acquired by John Wiley & Sons in February 2007. Blackwell's publishing programme has been merged with Wiley's global Scientific, Technical and Medical business to form Wiley-Blackwell.

Registered office: John Wiley & Sons Ltd, The Atrium, Southern Gate, Chichester, West Sussex, PO19 8SQ, UK

Editorial offices: 9600 Garsington Road, Oxford, OX4 2DQ, UK
      The Atrium, Southern Gate, Chichester, West Sussex, PO19 8SQ, UK
      111 River Street, Hoboken, NJ 07030-5774, USA

For details of our global editorial offices, for customer services and for information about how to apply for permission to reuse the copyright material in this book please see our website at www.wiley.com/wiley-blackwell

The right of the author to be identified as the author of this work has been asserted in accordance with the Copyright, Designs and Patents Act 1988.

Wiley also publishes its books in a variety of electronic formats. Some content that appears in print may not be available in electronic books.

Designations used by companies to distinguish their products are often claimed as trademarks. All brand names and product names used in this book are trade names, service marks, trademarks or registered trademarks of their respective owners. The publisher is not associated with any product or vendor mentioned in this book. This publication is designed to provide accurate and authoritative information in regard to the subject matter covered. It is sold on the understanding that the publisher is not engaged in rendering professional services. If professional advice or other expert assistance is required, the services of a competent professional should be sought.

The contents of this work are intended to further general scientific research, understanding, and discussion only and are not intended and should not be relied upon as recommending or promoting a specific method, diagnosis, or treatment by physicians for any particular patient. The publisher and the author make no representations or warranties with respect to the accuracy or completeness of the contents of this work and specifically disclaim all warranties, including without limitation any implied warranties of fitness for a particular purpose. In view of ongoing research, equipment modifications, changes in governmental regulations, and the constant flow of information relating to the use of medicines, equipment, and devices, the reader is urged to review and evaluate the information provided in the package insert or instructions for each medicine, equipment, or device for, among other things, any changes in the instructions or indication of usage and for added warnings and precautions. Readers should consult with a specialist where appropriate. The fact that an organization or Website is referred to in this work as a citation and/or a potential source of further information does not mean that the author or the publisher endorses the information the organization or Website may provide or recommendations it may make. Further, readers should be aware that Internet Websites listed in this work may have changed or disappeared between when this work was written and when it is read. No warranty may be created or extended by any promotional statements for this work. Neither the publisher nor the author shall be liable for any damages arising herefrom.

Library of Congress Cataloging-in-Publication Data

Endsley, D. Scott
  Putting healthcare innovation into practice / D. Scott Endsley.
    p. ; cm.
  Includes bibliographical references.
  ISBN 978-1-4443-3057-1
  1. Health services administration.   2. Medical care–Quality control.   3. Diffusion of innovations.   4. Health facilities–Administration.   5. Organizational change.   I. Title.
  [DNLM: 1. Health Facilities–organization & administration.   2. Organizational Innovation. WX 150 E56p 2010]
  RA399.A1E53 2010
  362.1068–dc22

                                     2009051155

ISBN: 9781444330571
A catalogue record for this book is available from the British Library.

Set in 9.25/12 pt Meridien by Aptara® Inc., New Delhi, India
Printed and bound in Singapore

1   2010

Contents

Foreword

In any business, leadership and innovation are essential to success in a competitive environment. We are particularly challenged in healthcare by the complex and often perverse payment and regulatory environment in which we operate. All too often, our mental models of what we have done in the past get in the way of thinking about how things could be in the future. To stay on top, healthcare organizations must constantly find new efficiencies while improving service, quality, and reliability.

Sustained organizational change takes real leadership. Creating and communicating a clear vision that all can understand begins the process of change. Everyone must be empowered to contribute in some way toward the desired future state. They must be able to see day-to-day progress in some meaningful way to stay engaged. This book will serve as a step-by-step guide to begin fostering a culture of innovation in your organization.

Healthcare organizations must intentionally instill a culture of improvement and innovation. It does not just happen by accident. Through a series of building blocks, tools, and scenarios, Dr Endsley has assembled a handy field guide to help your team develop a habit of idea generation and innovation. In succeeding chapters, you will see the importance of prototyping and testing ideas to make sure they work in the real world. Once these innovations have been tested, it is important to integrate and align promising new ideas throughout the organization.

Innovation in Action is the catalyst you need to get your people and your organization started on the important journey to a culture of improvement and innovation.

Bruce Bagley, MD
Past president, American Academy of Family Physicians
Medical Director for Quality for AAFP
February 2010

CHAPTER 1

Introduction to innovation

Welcome to *Innovation in Action*, a guidebook designed to provide insight, concepts, and tools for creating and testing new ideas (or redesigned old ideas) for healthcare. It is intended to help its users transform the practices and products that they use in their everyday delivery of healthcare and create value in the systems in which they work.

Tips for Innovation

1. Aim for simplicity
2. Think in verbs, not nouns
3. Build on ideas of others
4. Create an idea "treasure box"
5. Think both spatial as well as process change
6. Brainstorm often
7. Bring people together

What is innovation?

Innovation is "the first, practical, concrete implementation of an idea done in a way that brings broad-based, extrinsic recognition to an individual or organization."[1] Innovation goes beyond creativity, which is the production of ideas, to focus on implementation of ideas that bring value to individuals and organizations. It is a rare that innovations comes as "a bolt out of the blue" but more commonly, as Peter Drucker notes, are the result of "a conscious, purposeful search for innovation opportunities."[2] He emphasizes

---

Innovation in Action: A practical guide for healthcare teams, 1st edition.
By D. Scott Endsley. © 2010 Blackwell Publishing.

that innovation is a "systematic practice" that draws insights and ideas from interdisciplinary groups who see the innovation challenge from multiple perspectives. Unlike invention, innovation is first and foremost, a value-driven team set of processes with focused objectives.

> **Building Innovation into Health Systems: Memorial Hospital and Health System.** Memorial Hospital and Health Systems in South Bend, IN (*www.qualityoflife.org*), through senior leadership recognized that they were afflicted by a "creeping sameness," faced a war for talent, and were financially challenged by local competitors that were eating at their margins. Bringing innovation into their business model allowed them to all three of these. Leadership organized "innovisits" to regional organizations in and outside of healthcare recognized for their innovation (e.g., Proctor & Gamble), established board level policies that set expectations for innovation throughout the organization, created a system training program (Wizards College) in innovation for all level of staff, built innovation into job descriptions, and provided support through "idea propulsion labs" where "WoW projects were worked on." Memorial tracks costs and return on investments (ROI) for all innovation projects as a board expectation. ROI estimates range from 1.2 to 3.0 (120–300% return).

So why innovation? It is now acknowledged that the quality of healthcare in United States is average at best. For instance, a study by RAND[3] suggests that adults are receiving only 54.9% of recommended care (prevention, acute care, chronic services). "The need for change" as suggested by the RAND report "leads directly to the need for ideas for change."[4]

Innovation is distinctly different from invention—that is, the creation of something new. Innovation on the other hand requires that the new idea or creation is used and provides value to the users. It is fundamentally a team sport that involves people and ideas from multiple disciplines focused on an aim. As Peter Drucker has described it, innovation is a true discipline. Becoming an effective practitioner of innovation takes practice. As described by Peter Denning,[5] there are eight foundational practices for an innovator.

- *Awareness:* Ability to perceive opportunities, distinguishing them from your own agenda, ability to overcome cognitive blindness
- *Focus and persistence:* Ability to maintain attention on innovation challenge amidst chaos and obstacles
- *Listening and synthesizing:* Ability to hear others ideas, needs, preferences, and to blend them together with your own to create new ideas
- *Declarations:* Ability to make simple, powerful, moving, eloquent statements about the future that serve as attractors for others
- *Destiny:* A sense of the future and of possibilities that is powered by a larger purpose
- *Offers:* Bring value to your customers and stakeholders. Ability to deliver with commitment to results
- *Networks and allies:* Ability to build and maintain productive relationships with others, especially representing different perspectives and skills
- *Learning:* Constantly seeking new ideas, skills, and experiences from traditional and nontraditional sources; a mindset of inquiry

Beyond the distinction between innovation and invention, there are four myths about innovation of which to remain aware. These include (a) innovations must be big—often the most successful innovations are small, (b) innovations are the work of a gifted few—anyone can learn the skills and practice of innovation, (c) innovations are about new ideas—innovations are often old ideas in new uses or new audiences, and (d) innovations are only applicable to commercial markets—innovations are applicable in all settings (business, education, government, nonprofit, etc.).

Why is innovation so hard in healthcare

The United States spends over $26 billion on research and development in healthcare, second only to defense research and development.[6, 7] Yet examples of disastrous failures abound in healthcare—ranging from the various efforts to use managed care methods to manage costs, stock market losses of biotech start-ups, and the painfully slow digitalization of healthcare delivery—represent high stakes and high investment that yielded little in terms of innovations. Herzlinger[7] describes healthcare innovation in three sectors: consumer, technology, and business model.

She goes onto describe six forces that promote or kill innovation in healthcare. These are:

- *Players:* The diversity of stakeholders within healthcare is broad. Each has his or her own agendas and various degrees of influence on policymaking and resource allocation. Turf wars between hospitals and doctors and between consumers and health plans as well as other large and small battles compromise efforts to bridge differences and create space for innovation.

- *Funding:* Two financial challenges confront healthcare innovators. First, technology and pharmaceutical innovations require long lag times and rigorous Federal scrutiny before they are market ready. Second, the current reimbursement models are aimed at controlling cost, not supporting innovation. Insurers' benefit coverages are slow to integrate new technologies and innovations into their package of reimbursables.

- *Policy:* Healthcare is a highly regulated industry. These regulations can deter innovation development or dissemination of new technologies, drugs, or services. For example, the Stark Anti-Kickback statutes limited the ability of hospitals and affiliated office practices to collaborate on purchasing and supporting electronic health record systems.

- *Technology:* New technologies in healthcare are entering the market at lightning speed. Over the last 40 years, new technologies have accounted for 20–40% of the explosion of healthcare expenditures in the United States.[6] This "technological imperative," as Burns has described, is based on patient and provider demand for technologies that do not translate into healthcare value. Because of coverage and other issues, adoption of these technologies is highly variable, dependent on both market and interpersonal forces that are often difficult to predict with a particular technology. For instance, MRI scanners were highly market driven when introduced, leading to rapid uptake by the medical community. On the other hand, electronic information technologies are highly interpersonal driven, resulting in slower uptake.

- *Customers:* Over the last two decades, the role of the consumer has dramatically changed—from a passive, unknowing recipient of healthcare to a more active, informed manager of their own healthcare and healthcare dollars. For example, the rise of consumer-driven healthcare plans has ridden both the consumer's greater involvement and employers desire for lesser involvement. Direct-to-consumer marketing has changed the relationship between the patient and the provider, creating new opportunities for consumer-directed innovation.

- *Accountability:* Increasingly, healthcare providers, institutions, and payers are being held to standardized metrics of performance, often publicly reported. Moreover, these levels of performances are being incentivized through such programs at Bridges to Excellence or the Medicare Value-based purchasing initiatives. Thus, innovators are faced to helping potential users meet these performance demands.

These are the major forces with which the innovator must contend to be successful in bringing a creative idea to market and provide value to users.

Design thinking

Innovation is fundamentally a process of design. Specifically, innovation begins and ends with design for a user based on an understanding of the user's needs. It is differentiated from the practice of invention, in both being a team-based process and the primacy of the user in the design process. Figure 1.1 presents a model of design thinking and innovation developed by IDEO Inc.

Technological designers of products in healthcare start with optimizing feasibility of their product innovation, and then work on how to make it useful for people (desirability) and how to how to make a profit from their innovative product (viability). Business strategists design new business models and services and how to

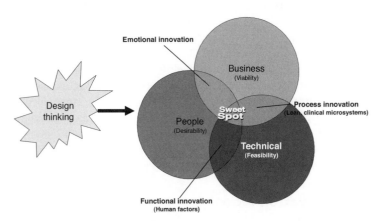

Figure 1.1 Model of design thinking.

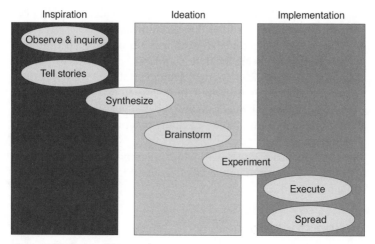

Figure 1.2 Phases of innovation.

effectively integrate technological tools into their offerings. Their focus is on "emotional innovation" or branding with a customer base.

Healthcare designers, on the other hand, start with what people need and desire, and then define the technical and/or service innovations that meet these needs. The approaches and tools described in Chapter 3 are geared to aiding the healthcare innovator to get into the heads, hearts, and lives of patients, caregivers, and providers in order to understand deeply where innovation might have the greatest impact (and market share). Healthcare organizations seeking to innovate often start at looking for the best ideas to prototype and take to market. There is a phase of innovation that precedes finding the best ideas that is finding inspiration through observation, inquiry, and storytelling that illuminates and informs the process of generating ideas (Figure 1.2). Once inspiration for innovation is discovered, the creative process of finding new ideas proceeds through synthesis of what is known, brainstorming ideas, and starting to experiment and prototype. Finally, as prototypes are tested, the usable/marketable form of the innovation emerges around which a business and marketing plan can be designed to expand the reach of the new product or service.

The innovation model

This guidebook is drawn from the work of IDEO, Inc, which is an internationally respected design firm headquartered in Palo

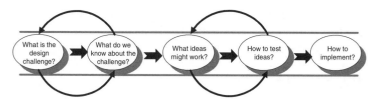

Figure 1.3 A model of innovation in action.

Alto, CA (see the IDEO website for information on their work: *www.ideo.com*). Considered one of the top 20 innovative companies in the world, IDEO devotes much of its corporate energy in assisting other companies develop a culture of innovation. This guidebook follows to an innovation model employed by IDEO[8] that includes a five-step process:

- Defining the innovation challenge
- Understanding the innovation challenge
- Generating innovative ideas
- Prototyping
- Making your innovation visible to others

This model suggests that the innovation process has its genesis in defining an existing or new need of a healthcare situation. A variety of tools and methods are then applied to examine the process and the user's experience of the process in order to better understand the needs of the user and the potential change points. This enhanced understanding of the innovation challenge generates new ideas to address the challenge from which the ideas with the highest potential are harvested and shaped into testable prototypes that can be experiential, mathematical, or physical (e.g., scale models). Rapid cycle testing of these prototypes allows the innovator to know if their idea would fly or not. If it would fly, the last step in the process is getting others inside and outside the organization to understand and support further development of the idea.

Although presented as a linear vector, these steps are often highly iterative. For instance, the prototyping and testing of an idea may generate a number of other, potentially better ideas. Or, in the process of assessing what is understood about an innovation challenge, there may be new questions about the aim or objective of the innovation.

This is a focused action model. It is not intended to portray the full lifecycle of an innovation that would also include organizational policy and leadership inputs, as well as a range of marketing strategies that would close the entrepreneurial loop.

Innovation teams

Innovations grow from a diversity of perspectives, knowledge, and experiences. In fact, innovation can be viewed as largely intersectional in which these different inputs are intermingled, producing an often unexpected array of new ideas, new products, and new services. The intersectional effect on innovation is called the Medici effect, first coined by Frans Johansson.[9]

As you organize for innovation in your workplace, put a team together that reflects a wide diversity of perspectives and backgrounds. These may be technicians, clinicians, administrators, clerical staff, and patients. Consider bringing in outside individuals who bring complementary perspective and skills such as people with communication expertise and marketing skills or individuals from other industries such as the hotel industry and manufacturing. For instance, Greater Ormond Hospital in London brought in race car pit crews to help them redesign their trauma services.

Tom Kelley from IDEO has proposed another way of thinking about diversity of innovation teams. He describe in his book, *The Ten Faces of Innovation*,[10] three major personas and 10 "faces" or personalities that invigorate the innovation process. Table 1.1 presents and describes these 10 faces. Kelley emphasizes that these are characteristics rather than characters: that is, that any one person can be any of the 10 faces over the course of time. He also emphasizes that not all 10 need be present on an innovation team to make it successful. Instead, the 10 faces approach is a guide for the type of roles that make innovation teams go.

An optimum team is 8–10 individuals with a team lead who plays the role of the director, and keeps the team on track and on schedule. Another myth of innovation is that it is about wild ideas and experimentation. It is, but is also about discipline, goals, and timelines.

Your innovation skills

As you prepare to engage in innovation in your work setting, how ready are you to be successful? An "innovation self-efficacy

Table 1.1 The 10 faces of innovation

Personas	Face	Description
Learning New Knowledge and Information	Anthropologist	Observes human behavior and understands how people interact with services, products, and physical spaces
	Experimenter	Prototypes and tries new ideas
	Cross-pollinator	An intersector (Medici effect) who brings different ideas from other cultures, organizations, and industries
Organizing Sets the stage and overcomes barriers	Hurdler	Overcomes barriers and constraints
	Collaborator	Brings people together, often with highly diverse perspectives, and acts as a mediator at times
	Director	Finds resources and keeps innovation team on track and on schedule
Building Apply ideas to organizations	Experience architect	Designs experiences that connect with people
	Set designer	Creates the stage on which the innovators work with attention to physical space and function
	Caregiver	Customer advocates who make sure team keeps needs and values of customer in the front and center of the innovation process
	Storyteller	Weaves the personal story around the innovation during the innovation process

Source: With permission from Reference 10.

assessment" is provided in Appendix A that gives you a sense of what innovation skills you possess and where there is opportunity to learn more. The 17 self-efficacy items are grouped into seven innovation categories including:

- Innovation team leadership
- Defining an innovation challenge
- Deep dive assessment
- Idea generation and selection
- Prototyping and testing
- Diffusion of innovations
- Innovation mentorship

Rate how confident you feel on these 17 innovation items on a scale of 1–10. Periodically, come back to this self-assessment and see how you are growing as an innovator.

Open innovation

Innovation is a team sport, requiring the inputs and insights from multiple perspectives including your customers. The broader the diversity of inputs, the more likely your innovation is to appeal to potential users. It is highly unlikely that you will have all the insights, knowledge, and skills to produce innovations on your own. Look for opportunity to collaborate across specialties, clinical units, organizations, or even economic domains.[11] The ability to bring cross-pollinator and collaborator skills to your innovation efforts will accelerate your ability to rapidly innovate in your organization.

Open innovation is a rapidly growing business model in other economic sectors. For instance, Proctor & Gamble has developed an initiative called Connect and Develop. P&G has an extensive network of innovation scouts that find small companies developing products. P&G provides capital, licenses, or purchases these products, and then takes them to market (the best example is the Swiffer brush).

In healthcare, open models have been used in quality collaboratives[12] and more recently in learning networks. For example, the Innovation Learning Network (ILN) is a cooperative of large healthcare organizations (see Figure 1.3) that work together both in person and remotely on innovating on common issues for member organizations. They have developed an open innovation toolkit that can be found at ***iln-public.pbwiki.com/2006ILNLearnings***.

An innovation story: Greenfield Health System

Stories are often an effective way of learning how innovation strategies can be applied in real world settings. Throughout this guidebook, you will find illuminating examples of how healthcare organizations have tackled innovation challenges in their environment.

Starting below, you will also find a synthetic story of a made-up healthcare organization, and how they applied innovation principles and methods to integrating innovation into their daily work. This story will successively unfold across the chapters to illustrate applications of the methods described in the chapter.

Greenfield Health Systems is a small physician-hospital organization that is composed of a 220-bed community hospital and a physician network of 80 physicians in 24 practices, both single and multispecialty. Greenfield has been actively involved with improvement efforts, including participation in the Institute for Healthcare Improvement's 5 Million Lives Campaign. The Chief Executive Officer, Mr Seawright, in consultation with the Chief Nursing Officer, Ms Highcare, has concluded that the health reform pressures from Washington will require them to become more nimble for change and more efficient in delivering care. They realized that they needed to be more "innovative" in the services and business strategies that they use. Ms Highcare identifies a nurse on 4E who seems to have a bent for doing things differently, and has designed a number of new ways of working on the unit. This nurse is appointed the "head" of a new innovation team, with representatives from the medical staff, pharmacy, ancillary services, and administration. Although from diverse backgrounds and with different agendas, this team feels empowered by the CEO and the health system board.

How to use this guidebook

This guidebook is organized based on the five steps of the innovation process outlined in the model above. Each chapter is dedicated to a step in the process and offers selected tools to go through the step. Every chapter has (a) an overview of the innovation step, (b) a tool package useful for the step, and (c) a set of resources. In addition, an example healthcare organization confronting an innovation challenge is presented that is used to illustrate the core activities for each innovation step.

This guidebook is not intended to be read at a single setting, but to provide ideas and tools based on the starting point of the user. These steps are however linked, and should be seen as a high-level "system" of innovation processes that will get more efficient with practice.

You are encouraged to read, digest, and try the processes and tools described in each chapter. You are encouraged as well to adapt and disseminate any of the tools, models, or examples used in this guide. Our goal is to provide a learning catalyst that enables you to become an effective innovator in your healthcare organization.

Good luck on your journey!

Appendix A: clinical innovation self-efficacy

We would like to know how confident you are in doing certain activities. For each of the following questions, please choose the number that corresponds to your confidence that you can do the tasks regularly at the present time.

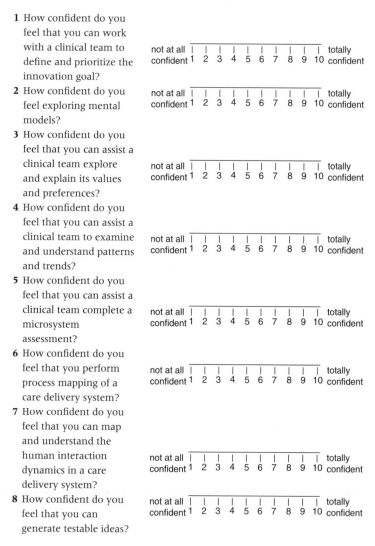

1 How confident do you feel that you can work with a clinical team to define and prioritize the innovation goal?

not at all confident 1 2 3 4 5 6 7 8 9 10 totally confident

2 How confident do you feel exploring mental models?

not at all confident 1 2 3 4 5 6 7 8 9 10 totally confident

3 How confident do you feel that you can assist a clinical team explore and explain its values and preferences?

not at all confident 1 2 3 4 5 6 7 8 9 10 totally confident

4 How confident do you feel that you can assist a clinical team to examine and understand patterns and trends?

not at all confident 1 2 3 4 5 6 7 8 9 10 totally confident

5 How confident do you feel that you can assist a clinical team complete a microsystem assessment?

not at all confident 1 2 3 4 5 6 7 8 9 10 totally confident

6 How confident do you feel that you perform process mapping of a care delivery system?

not at all confident 1 2 3 4 5 6 7 8 9 10 totally confident

7 How confident do you feel that you can map and understand the human interaction dynamics in a care delivery system?

not at all confident 1 2 3 4 5 6 7 8 9 10 totally confident

8 How confident do you feel that you can generate testable ideas?

not at all confident 1 2 3 4 5 6 7 8 9 10 totally confident

9 How confident do you feel that you can lead a brainstorming session?

not at all confident | 1 2 3 4 5 6 7 8 9 10 | totally confident

10 How confident do you feel that you can select an idea to test?

not at all confident | 1 2 3 4 5 6 7 8 9 10 | totally confident

11 How confident do you feel that you can build a material prototype including scale models?

not at all confident | 1 2 3 4 5 6 7 8 9 10 | totally confident

12 How confident do you feel that you can build a mathematical prototype?

not at all confident | 1 2 3 4 5 6 7 8 9 10 | totally confident

13 How confident do you feel that you can organize and conduct an experience prototype?

not at all confident | 1 2 3 4 5 6 7 8 9 10 | totally confident

14 How confident do you feel that you can find or design performance measures as element of test?

not at all confident | 1 2 3 4 5 6 7 8 9 10 | totally confident

15 How confident do you feel that you can present results of prototype test using a storyboard?

not at all confident | 1 2 3 4 5 6 7 8 9 10 | totally confident

16 How confident do you feel that you understand dissemination (diffusion) strategies for broad implementation of an idea?

not at all confident | 1 2 3 4 5 6 7 8 9 10 | totally confident

17 How confident do you feel that you can teach and assist others in performing innovation activities?

not at all confident | 1 2 3 4 5 6 7 8 9 10 | totally confident

Scoring

The score for each item is the number circled. If two consecutive numbers are circled, code the lower number (less self-efficacy). If the numbers are not consecutive, do not score the item. The score for the scale is the mean of the 17 items. If more than 2 items are missing, do not score the scale. Higher number indicates higher self-efficacy.

References

1. Plsek PE. *Creativity, Innovation, and Quality*, ASQ Quality Press, Milwaukee, WI, 1997.
2. Drucker PF. "The Discipline of Innovation," *Harvard Business Review*, August 2002.
3. McGlynn EA, Asch SM, Adams J, Keesey J, Hicks J, DeCristofaro A, Kerr EA. "The Quality of Healthcare Delivered to Adults in the United States," *New England Journal of Medicine*, 2003, **348**(26), 2635–2645.
4. Plsek P. "Innovative Thinking for the Improvement of Medical Systems," *Annals of Internal Medicine*, 1999, **131**, 438–444.
5. Denning PJ. "The Social Life of Innovation," *Communications of the ACM*, 2004, **47**(4), 15–19.
6. Burns LR. *The Business of Healthcare Innovation*, Cambridge University Press, Cambridge, UK, 2006.
7. Herzlinger RE. "Why Innovation in Healthcare Is So Hard," *Harvard Business Review*, May 2006.
8. Nussbaum B. "The Power of Design," *BusinessWeek*, May 17, 2004.
9. Johansson F. *The Medici Effect: What Elephants and Epidemics Can Teach Us About Innovation*, Harvard Business School Press, Boston, 2006.
10. Kelley T. *The Ten Faces of Innovation*, Doubleday, New York, 2005.
11. Chesbrough H. *Open Business Models: How to Thrive in the New Innovation Landscape*, Harvard Business School Press, Boston, 2006.
12. Kilo CM. "A Framework for Collaborative Improvement: Lessons from the Institute for Healthcare Improvement's Breakthrough Series," *Quality Management in Healthcare*, 1998, **6**(4), 1–13.

CHAPTER 2
Defining the innovation challenge

Innovation is a purpose-driven, team-based, systematic set of activities whose goal is to bring value to individuals and organizations. As you approach innovation, a key first step is to define where you want to focus and why it is important to work in this area. This step cannot be emphasized enough if often neglected in the innovation process. The best ideas without a purpose or direction are simply good ideas. Most innovation solutions fail,[1] with only 4.5% succeeding in the marketplace. Much of this high failure rate can be attributed to poorly framed innovation challenges.[2] Remember, the goal of your innovation work should be not to have the best ideas, but to have the best ideas that bring value to you or your organization. Value is defined at this step in the process.

The opportunities for innovation come from a variety of sources. Peter Drucker in his foundational work, *Innovation and Entrepreneurship*,[3] identified eight sources from which innovation opportunities arise which include:

- Unexpected successes or failures
- Incongruities—a gap between reality and common belief
- Process need—a bottleneck in a critical process
- Change of industry structure—new business models, distribution channels, and modes of business
- Demographics—changes in groups by age, politics, religion, income, etc.
- Change of mood or perception—change in the way people see the world (e.g., post 9/11)

Innovation in Action: A practical guide for healthcare teams, 1st edition.
By D. Scott Endsley. © 2010 Blackwell Publishing.

- New knowledge—application of new knowledge, involving scientific advances and convergences
- Marginal practices—fringe practices that may resolve gaps or failures of the current process

Selection of the greatest innovation challenge is impacted by the following factors:

External mandates. These include what healthcare payers and employers may be demanding (e.g., improvement in access to care) or may reflect national mandates emanating from the bodies such as the Institute of Medicine or the National Quality Forum. Finally, they may also be the result of Federal requirements, such as those captured in the Medicare Modernization Act or legislation from Congress.

Requirements/needs/preferences of users. Healthcare organizations and their providers and staffs may have definable needs and requirements that call for innovation products or services: for example, a hospital that need tools to improve blood loss during specific types of surgery, or unit staff who need more effective ways of managing the distribution of medications, or an emergency department that need to decompress the workflows during peak hours.

Gaps in care (quality/access). Data from local and national sources may be invaluable in defining where the greatest gaps in care exist and the specific factors that contribute to the gaps. For example, the author conducted a logistic analysis of data on low birth weight infants in Missouri, and identified domestic abuse as a strong predictor in this population of a low birth weight delivery. Subsequently, an initiative was designed to train OB providers on the use of the ACOG (American College of Obstetricians and Gynecologists) domestic violence screening tool, and open access to women's shelters.

Potential for impact. Understanding the epidemiologic patterns and clinical logic of a health condition may identify points where new strategies may most effectively improve outcomes. For instance, innovations that enhance the likelihood of a patient with coronary artery disease risk factors to engage in behavioral risk reduction activities are more likely to decrease cardiovascular mortality than interventions targeted at later stages of the disease (e.g., angioplasty).

The tools and methods discussed in this chapter are designed to assist you and your innovation team in identifying where the innovation challenges lie, and to help you prioritize candidate areas for innovation work.

> **The Productive Ward and Redesign of Patient Transport.** The UK National Institute for Innovation and Improvement is the central support center for innovation across the National Health Service (***www.institute.nhs.uk***). The Institute has developed programs and tools for clinical providers to improve care delivery and outcomes of care. One program, The Productive Ward, aimed to redesign care in inpatient units to allow nursing staff greater time to provide care. The Institute held focus groups of clinical providers and auxiliary staff to determine where to start. One core area that many participants identified as a constraint to efficient care delivery was transport of patients. The Institute then brought together select porters (orderlies) to investigate and redesign the function of porter-assisted transport. The redesign effort led to a prototype that included a "porter central" that allowed better management of assignment and flow of porters through the hospital.

A strategy for defining the innovation challenge

Finding and framing innovation challenges can be laborious (but important) work. Figure 2.1 presents a strategy to getting a well-framed innovation challenge that informs the deep dive and prototyping process. It includes:

- Interviewing management, frontline staff, and patients/customers of the organization
- Reviewing organizational reports and data
- Searching through literature, online sources, and external contacts for information on the area
- Identifying the priority theme

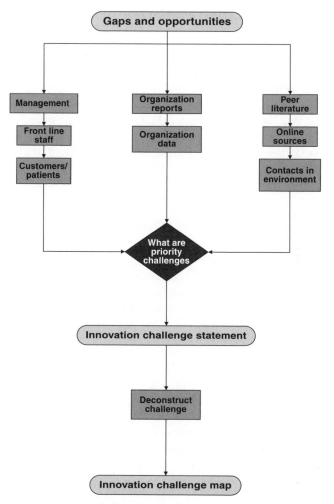

Figure 2.1 Innovation challenge process.

- Framing the theme as a challenge statement
- Optionally deconstructing the challenge statement into associated elements by management, frontline, and patient perspectives
- Mapping these elements to further refine the starting point and value of the to be developed innovation solution

Step 1: information gathering

360° *interviews*

Interviews with managers, frontline staff, and patients or customers can illuminate the gaps and desires for innovation. Interviews can focus on where the current service or products fall short of expectation (*looking for problems*) or can focus on where there is a strong current foundation upon which to build our potential future dreams and directions (*looking for promise*). Both are important in better understanding the innovation opportunities in your organization or the healthcare environment.

Tool 1: question databank

Description

A list of questions framed to elicit knowledge and perspectives from management, frontline staff, and patients or customers. These allow a more structured way to collect useful information that can identify themes for innovation. Questions can be both problem identification and strength identification. See Appendix A for an example question bank.

Use

Arrange 30 minutes with selected management, frontline staff, and patients. Two to four interviews per category are a reasonable start to provide a representative series of perspectives. Ask the appropriate type of question for the interviewee (e.g., financial questions for managers and experience of care questions for patients). Record themes on Innovation Challenge form (see Appendix B).

Tool 2: discovery interviews

Description

Design challenges are often based on real or perceived deficits in service or performance. As noted above, gap analysis can help clarify where the greatest opportunities for innovation may lie. Equally important, however, is the exploration of the aspects of healthcare that care providers and patients experience in the delivery process, especially those aspects that bring delight and satisfaction to the

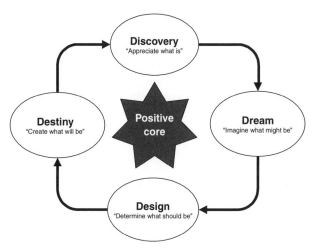

Figure 2.2 Appreciative inquiry cycle.
(used with permission of author)

users.[4] Discovery interviews are rooted in the work of appreciative inquiry.[5] Discovery is the first of the four D's, and involves interviews with users of the healthcare system, service, or product, and is focused on eliciting their experiences, particularly those that highlight the positives (see Figure 2.2).

Use
1. Identify the users to interview
2. Construct the interview guide
3. Conduct the interviews
4. Analyze the themes that emerge
5. Group themes into affinity groups

Users chosen should reflect the full spectrum of the experience. These should include patients and families, physicians and nursing staff, and other professional staff.

The interview guide should be a brief, one-page outline of key questions. The questions should be open-ended and solicit the "stories" of the users. For example, some questions might be:

Tell me what it is like being a [patient, provider] . . .

What do you value most about being a [patient, provider] at this. . .

What do you find unique about being a [patient, provider] at this...

Describe your best experience being a [patient, provider] at this...

If you had three wishes to make this a better experience as a [patient, provider], what would they be?

If you could redesign one aspect of this experience as a [patient, provider], what would you redesign?

In five years, this [name of healthcare setting or service] is being honored for its excellence, why?

Arrange for a specific time and place to conduct the Discovery Interview. Begin by introducing the purpose of the interview and offer an invitation to their stories. Ask about their general experience for focus on what brings value and delight. Ask additional, deeper questions around themes that are raised. For example, "tell me more how you get timely and useful information from your doctor." Write down statements as close to verbatim as possible.

After each interview, summarize what you identify as being the themes you detect and get feedback from the interviewee. Following completion of the Discovery Interviews, list all the themes that have emerged across the interviews.

Resources
The Institute for Innovation and Improvement of the National Health Service in the United Kingdom has produced a guide to conducting Discovery Interviews that can be found at ***www.institute .nhs.uk/index.php?option=com_joomcart&Itemid=194&main_page =document_product_info&products_id=269.***

Information search
An important complement to interviews is review and distillation of information from within your own organization as well as from outside organizations, and from the literature.

Information from own organization
Identify recent performance reports from your organization. These may be self-generated or provided by health plans with which the organization contracts. What are the major themes needing improvement? What are the major themes demonstrating excellence? Are there trends or patterns?

Information from outside organizations

Talk with colleagues in other healthcare organizations. Review summary reports from national organizations that monitor trends in quality and utilization performance. Examples include:

Commonwealth Fund
Chartbooks/Chartpack: ***www.commonwealthfund.org/***
Agency for Healthcare Research and Quality (AHRQ) national quality
   reports:
   – National Healthcare Quality Report
   – National Healthcare Disparity Report
   – Both at ***http://www.ahrq.gov/qual/measurix.htm***
Institute for the Future produces forecasts for healthcare as well as a
   series of reports focusing on leading edge issues affecting societal
   change that impacts delivery of healthcare.
   – Health   and   Healthcare   2010:   ***www.iftf.org/system/files/***
      deliverables/SR-794_Health_%2526_Health_Care_2010.pdf
   – Expanded   Meanings   of   Health: ***www.iftf.org/system/files/***
      deliverables/SR-815B_Meanings_of_Health.pdf
   – Top   Ten   Impediments   to   Better   Health   and   Health-
      care: ***www.iftf.org/system/files/deliverables/SR-900_Top_Ten_***
      Impediments.pdf
   – Personal   Health   Ecologies: ***www.iftf.org/system/files/***
      deliverables/SR_876A_Personal_Health_Ecologies.pdf
Institute of Medicine's healthcare quality reports provide insightful
   summaries of issues and solutions facing healthcare. The Quality
   of Healthcare in America project at Institute of Medicine produced a series of reports including Crossing the Quality Chasm:
   www.iom.edu/en/Reports/2001/Crossing-the-Quality-Chasm-A-
   New-Health-System-for-the-21st-Century.aspx
Rand Corp. produces a wide variety of in-depth, well-researched reports with data summaries, which can be found at **http://rand.**
   org/health/

Tool 3: scenario planning

Description

Beyond looking at past performance and trends as well as current status and needs, it can be illuminating to consider the possible future scenarios for your organization and for healthcare.
Scenario planning is widely used in Europe, which is led by Royal
Dutch/Shell, and is the centerpiece of future thinking process.

Use

1. Identify a team of eight to ten individuals with knowledge and expertise in your organization or in the topic of focus. This team should have not only clinicians but also administrators, information technology and finance experts, and executive leadership

2. Propose a focus for the scenario, and facilitate a discussion (an hour is usually sufficient) on the definition and nature of the proposed focus. Examples might include:
   (a) transitioning care from the hospital to the community
   (b) automation of the clinical process
   (c) direct contracting with consumers

3. Brainstorm a list of key factors that might affect the future scenario. Spend 1–3 hours in active brainstorming, looking for 50–100 key factors. Driving forces can be:
   (a) social forces
   (b) technological forces
   (c) economic forces
   (d) environmental factors
   (e) political forces

4. Label each of these factors/forces as predetermined, which are trends already in progress, or critical uncertainties, which are forces that may significantly change the nature of the future scenario

5. Group the factors by common themes

6. Identify the two themes that seem to be the most critical, define the extreme ends of the theme, and lay them out in a matrix (see example in Figure 2.3)

7. Divide into two to four subteams and spend 1 hour writing the outlines of a "story" for each quadrant of the matrix, and then have each team present the scenario for the quadrant to the whole group. These should be stories that have characters, plots, and endings. Look 5–20 years into the future

8. Discuss and identify as a group the areas where innovation might accelerate positive impacts or minimize negative impacts

Resources

The Global Innovation Network is an international business consulting organization that grew out of the Royal Dutch/Shell experience with scenario planning. They have produced a guide to scenario planning called "Plotting Your Scenarios" available at *www.gbn.com*. Martin Börjesson, a European futurist, has created

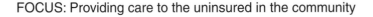

FOCUS: Providing care to the uninsured in the community

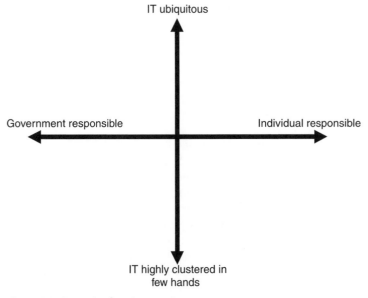

Figure 2.3 Scenario planning matrix.

a resource Web site for scenario planning that provides tools and information on conducting scenario planning exercises. It is available at *www.well.com/~mb/scenario_planning/*. ScenarioThinking.org is a wiki Web site devoted to scenario planning, and provides for online, collaborative scenario writing. It is available at *scenariothinking.org/wiki/index.php/Main_Page*.

Data analysis
If time and facility exist, examining data from your institution may illuminate innovation challenges. Analysis may range from hand calculation of counts to more advanced statistical evaluation of multifactorial associations.

Tool 4: data analysis and review

Description
As a complement to experience-based and value-oriented user explorations, it is often helpful to examine what data and information

are available about the characteristics of the organization under study and how it is performing. Often information is already available that may inform your choice of innovation challenge, or you may need to do some brief analysis of existing data sets.

Use
1. Identify sources of information and data
2. Review and summarize the key findings
3. Conduct brief analysis as needed
4. Present findings to group
5. Discuss where gaps may be found
6. Use nominal group techniques to group and prioritize

Useful sources of information include financial reports and data, user surveys, public health reports, reports produced by the parent organization, and performance reports from health plans and payers. Further information may be gleaned from basic analyses of available, organization-specific data sets.

Based on available information, identify where there are opportunities for innovation (e.g., target audience, service line, healthcare function, products and other tools that are or could be used).

Step 2: prioritization

In Step 1, you gather information from interviews, environmental scan, review of organization data, and possibly some data analysis that you have captured on the Innovation Challenge Statement & Strategy Map form (see Appendix B). Now you need to pick a starting point for your innovation work. Working with your innovation team, you can select your priority focus on initiating your innovation work. To start with, list the themes you have discovered in Step 1 on a large Post-It or white board, and then apply the nominal group technique as described in Tool 5.

Tool 5: nominal group technique

Description
The nominal group technique (NGT) is a method of soliciting pooled judgments from the innovation team (and other stakeholders). It involves four types of procedures: generating ideas, recording ideas,

discussing ideas, and voting on ideas. The last three procedures are useful for ideas generated from other approaches (discovery interviews, gap analysis, etc.).

Use
1. Group members write topic ideas for innovation challenges silently and independently. Allow adequate time
2. The group facilitator writes the topics idea of a group member on a flipchart and proceeds to ask next group member, and so on. Important to number the idea. Allow the member to "pass" if there are no new ideas. Record rapidly in exact works. Discussion and debate not allowed at this point
3. Group discusses each idea in turn specifically to clarify topic idea and understand logic behind innovation topic. Facilitator groups ideas based on consensus
4. Each group member is allowed to multivote. Use colored dots (e.g., five per member), and allow each member to place next to topic idea(s) they feel merit focus. Continue for additional rounds to narrow the topics to one priority topic (overwhelming majority of dots)

Resources
The University of Wisconsin has developed an NGT user's guide that is helpful in organizing and conducting NGT sessions available at *http://www.peoplemix.com/documents/general/ngt.pdf.*

The Centers for Disease Control and Prevention also have a brief guide to nominal group sessions available at *www.cdc.gov/HealthyYouth/evaluation/pdf/brief7.pdf*

Step 3: writing your innovation statement

Based on the priority innovation challenge identified in Step 2, it is critical to capture it in a way that informs and guides subsequent innovation work, especially your deep dive. Using Appendix B, write down your topic area and frame the innovation challenge starting with "How might we. . . ." A well-configured innovation challenge statement will have a single objective, avoids leaping to preconceived solutions or evaluation criteria, and is "smart."

Tool 6: smart innovation challenges

Description
It has been said that "if you don't [know] where you are going, then you won't know when you get there." Setting a clear innovation statement helps you clarify the terrain where you will explore for innovation.

A workable innovation challenge has a set of smart characteristics. As you consider and formulate your innovation, make them specific, measurable, attributable, relevant, and time-framed.

Use
1. Identify priority theme based on Step 2
2. Frame the theme in actionable terms with smart characteristics
3. Key is enough specificity to provide initial direction and position of the innovation work within a setting or patient population, etc., and enough breadth to provide flexibility in innovation solution

Note: Do not lock yourself too early into a solution.

Resources
A number of excellent project planning tools exist. The Institute for Healthcare Improvement offers guidance and tips for aims setting available at *www.ihi.org/IHI/Topics/Improvement/Improvement Methods/HowToImprove/setting+aims.htm.*

Step 4: mapping your innovation strategy

Your Innovation Challenge Statement may provide enough direction to get started with the deep dive. If not, an innovation strategy map may help you find the right level of challenge (see Figure 2.4).

Tool 7: innovation strategy map

Description
A visual representation of innovation challenge objectives by location within a healthcare setting (e.g., management, frontline, and patient), which allows determination of which objectives are the primary constraints where innovation efforts might bear the most fruit.

Innovation Challenge Statement

How might we make it easier for a nurse to administer medications to patients in a safe and timely manner

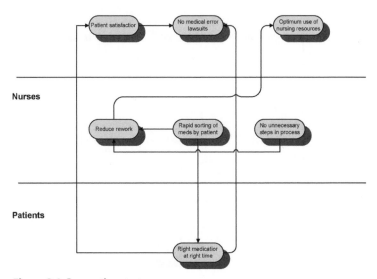

Figure 2.4 Innovation strategy map.

Use

1. List all the objectives for each level (management, frontline, patient) for the innovation challenge as captured in the Innovation Challenge Statement
2. Graph these objectives at their appropriate level on the Innovation Strategy Map (see Appendix B)
3. Connect these objectives together based on which require or impact other objectives (see Figure 2.5)
4. Determine which objectives have the greatest number of inbound or outbound connections: nodes with the greatest inbound connections represent the constraining factors in the system; nodes with the greatest outbound connections represent the factors with the greatest influence. Quality improvement strategies tend to focus on mitigating constraints in processes and systems. Innovation strategies work best on the nodes that emanate the greatest influence

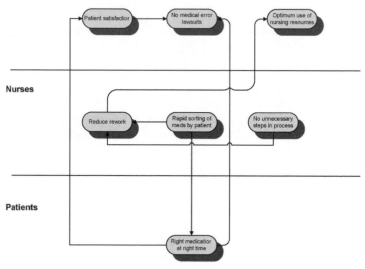

Innovation Challenge Statement

How might we make it easier for a nurse to administer medications to patients in a safe and timely manner

Figure 2.5 Example strategy map.

5. Be prepared to redraw your map as you begin your exploration. You may discover new nodes and connections as you do your deep dive

Resource
The Innovation Strategy Map as described above is taken from Van Gundy's white paper 'Care and Framing of Strategic Innovation Challenges' available at - ***www.jpb.com/creative/VanGundy FrameInnov.pdf.***

An innovation story continued

The Greenfield innovation team begins their collective work by gathering reports and information not only about Greenfield Health Systems but also from regional competitors and reform white papers from Washington. They comb these reports for areas where innovation might be needed as well as those areas where Greenfield Health Systems does well. The team also splits ups and interviews using a structured form the head nurses and physician unit directors on all the floors of the hospital, as well as the major ambulatory centers. They also interview health system leadership including the CEO, CNO, Chair, Board of Directors, Quality and Risk Management directors, and Pharmacy director.

During an innovation team meeting, the team put up all the topics that bubbled up during the literature review and structured interviews on an easel board for discussion. These were grouped by theme, and each committee member silently prioritized the top three using a nominal method. The leading area for innovation was prioritized by this method as the discharge process. Specifically, the team identified high rates of readmissions that were felt to be related to inadequate discharge and follow-up processes of care. Subsequently, the team undertook a focused literature search on improvement strategies for discharge and prevention of readmissions.

Appendix A: Innovation challenge question bank

1. What does our organization do?
2. What does our organization want to do in the future?
3. Who are our patients/customers?
4. Who would we like to have as customers?
5. How do our patients/customers see us?
6. What services/products do we offer that we think are successful (and why)?
7. What services/products we offer that we think are unsuccessful (an why)?
8. What are the trends in the healthcare market?
9. What are our biggest headaches in our work?
10. What are our biggest rewards in our work?
11. What three things—services or products—would help us excel?

Appendix B: Innovation Challenge Statement & Strategy Map

Submitted by: _____

Instructions: Based on your interviews with Executive Management, frontline staff, and patients, and based on information you have through review of the literature and external sources, define the key strategic challenges for a topic area from the viewpoints of management, staff, and patients/customers. Then connect them together. See attached example.

What I learned from discussions with management

Discussion themes:

What I learned from discussions with frontline staff

Discussion themes:

What I learned from discussions with patients or customers

Discussion themes:

What I learned from review of reports, literature, data, environmental scan

Evidence themes:

My Innovation Challenge Statement

Innovation   **Topic**   **Area:**

Innovation Challenge Statement:

How might we:

_____

_____

_____

_____

_____

e.g. How might we make it easier for a nurse to administer the correct medications to a patient in a timely and safe manner?

My Innovation Strategy Map

Management

_____

Frontline Staff

_____

Patients/Customers

_____

> Innovation
> Objective

References

1. Nussbaum B. "The Power of Design," *BusinessWeek*, found at: *http://www.ideo.com/images/uploads/thinking/publications/pdfs/power_of_design.pdf*.
2. Van Gundy, AB. "The Care and Framing of Strategic Innovation Challenges," *www.jpb.com/creative/VanGundyFrameInnov.pdf*.
3. Drucker P. *Innovation and Entrepreneurship*, Harper Publishing, New York, 1985.
4. Bate P, Robert G. "Experience-based Design: From Redesigning the System Around the Patient to Co-Designing Services with the Patient," *Quality & Safety in Healthcare*, 2006, **15**, 307–310.
5. Whitney D, Trosten-Bloom A. *The Power of Appreciative Inquiry: A Practice Guide for Positive Change*, Berrett-Koehler Publishers, San Francisco, CA, 2003.

CHAPTER 3

The deep dive

Once you have defined the innovation challenge, the next step is to understand the challenge as comprehensively as possible. Key to this process is using techniques to explore the experiences, needs, and opportunities of users ("hitting the streets" as IDEO likes to say). IDEO has adapted a panel of methods from anthropology and the social sciences to enable a "deep dive" into the innovation challenge. IDEO categorizes these strategies into four main types (Figure 3.1):

Learn refers to collecting, synthesizing, and analyzing available information about the innovation challenge. This may include reports and studies both in the published and in the gray literature. It also includes not only information specifically about the topic but other related areas such as community served, evidence on procedures and technologies, human resources, and other areas.

Look includes a variety of observation methods to capture the experience of users impacted by the innovation challenge. These include behavioral observation and mapping of patterns, rituals, and artifacts, photo or video surveys, and process mapping.

Ask encompasses an array of techniques to elicit information from users and others. These include focus and unfocus groups, activity analysis surveys, knowledge–attitude–practice (KAP) surveys, mind mapping, and bodystorming.

Try is a learning process by doing. Building physical, mathematical, performance prototypes not only captures your innovative idea for others to see and test, but also allows the designer the chance to "build to think," as Tim Brown, the CEO at IDEO, has said.[1] Prototyping, trying something out, is a way of unlocking the intuitions of innovation teams, and allows new knowledge about underlying assumptions.

Innovation in Action: A practical guide for healthcare teams, 1st edition.
By D. Scott Endsley. © 2010 Blackwell Publishing.

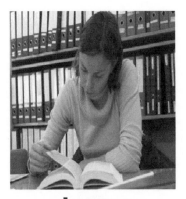

Learn

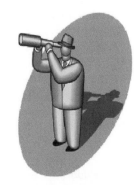

Look

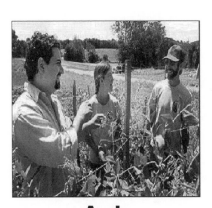

Ask

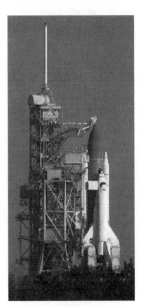

Try

Figure 3.1 IDEO four strategies.

Nurse Knowledge Exchange at Kaiser Permanente.
Kaiser Permanente has established an internal "innovation
consultancy" (*xnet.kp.org/innovationcenter/*) based at the
Garfield Innovation Center in San Leandro, California. Spurred
by the system roll out of an electronic health record, the
innovation consultancy was engaged to redesign workflows to
take advantage of electronic flow of health information in four
hospitals representing four of Kaiser Permanente California
regions. Exchange of patient information at shift change
for nurses arose as a key priority for redesign. Extensive review
of the literature was conducted and national experts consulted.
Stories were collected from the frontlines and shared with the
innovation team. Nurses were shadowed and observed, and focus groups were held with nurses, physicians, and pharmacists
who were asked to draw the process of shift change.

The tools and methods described below are a small selection of a
broad array of strategies to dive into your innovation topic. You are
encouraged to explore others as you learn them, and bring them
back to your innovation team.

A valuable resource in this effort is the IDEO Method Cards (see
article for description of IDEO Method Cards at *www.fastcompany.
com/magazine/75/outofthebox.html*). IDEO has captured 51 strategies for learning, looking, asking, and trying that can be selected.
They serve as references and prompts in the deep dive innovation
assessment process. More information on the method cards can be
found at *http://www.ideo.com/work/item/method-cards/*.

Learn

These tools help you acquire knowledge about the challenge that
others have learned. These sources include gathering information
from published and unpublished literature, online sites, and organizational documents and reports.

Tool 1: PubMed search

Description
PubMed is the National Library of Medicine database and search
engine that contains a comprehensive listing of published literature

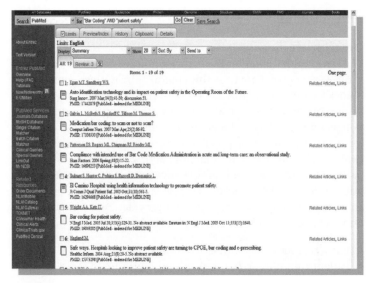

Figure 3.2 PubMed.

that can be searched using a lexicon of keywords and string operators. Searches can be narrowed using user-selected filters. Many of the search results provide full-text abstracts and articles (Figure 3.2).

Use

1. Enter the URL in your browser ***www.ncbi.nlm.nih.gov/sites/ entrez***
2. Type in your keyword and operators as needed
3. Click on "Limits" to set filter parameters (e.g., English only)
4. View search results
5. Click on specific search result to view abstract
6. Click in "box" to select document for search set
7. On the bottom bar, select file under "send to" to produce a bibliographic document that you can print

Resources

The National Library of Medicine offers a free online tutorial on use of PubMed that can be found at ***www.nlm.nih.gov/bsd/ pubmed_tutorial/m1001.html***. A primer on use of PubMed can be found at ***http://nnlm.gov/training/resources/pmtri.pdf***.

Tool 2: clinical microsystems

Description

The Dartmouth Center for Evaluative Clinical Sciences has designed a redesign toolkit based on the clinical microsystem model. This model focuses on the interaction between the patient and a small system of physicians, nurses, administrative support, and information technology all linked together for the specific purpose of caring for a specific patient or population of patients. It recognizes that healthcare is delivered by small, dynamic communities of clinical practice where innovation and change are catalyzed. The clinical microsystem model proposes that assessment (diagnosis) of the microsystem encompasses the 5 P's and provides a set of data collection and analysis tools for each P (Figure 3.3):

- Purpose: motivators/attractors for health unit
- Patients: number, types, satisfaction with care, disease distribution
- Professionals: composition of providers, their full-time equivalent, and their skills and capacity

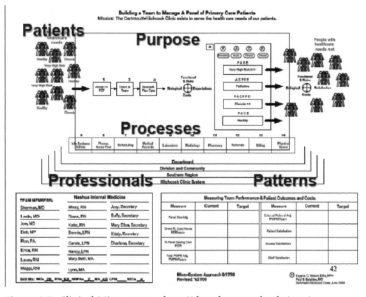

Figure 3.3 Clinical Microsystem. *http://dms.dartmouth.edu/cms/*

- Processes: demand for services, work efficiency (time hand-offs), constraints, and bottlenecks
- Patterns: trends in outcomes and financial performance

Use
1. Organize a lead team – include representatives from the different components of the microsystem: physicians, nurses, clerks, support staff
2. Assess the 5 P's
3. Make a diagnosis
4. Treat the microsystem
5. Follow-up

The workbooks for outpatient primary care, outpatient specialty care, emergency department, and inpatient units provide a compilation of tools to evaluate the five P's.

These include:

Patients
- Access to care survey
- Patient viewpoint (experience of care) survey
- Through the eyes of your patients walk-through
- Assessment of care for chronic conditions survey

Professionals
- Staff satisfaction survey
- Staff skills assessment
- Practice activity survey

Processes
- Patient visit cycle time survey
- Core and supporting processes evaluation
- Process mapping tool

Patterns
- Unplanned activity tracking card
- Telephone tracking log

Data from the 5-P evaluation are used to determine where processes are underperforming, producing hassles and dissatisfaction among staff and patients, subject to undue waits and delays, and are a source of wide variation.

Treatment of the healthcare unit involves creating or adapting innovations to test using rapid cycle tests of change. Microsystem models propose that innovations fall into four categories: changes in access to care and information, changes in interactions, changes in reliability of care delivery, and changes that enhance vitality of the organization.

Resources
Dartmouth makes available a downloadable microsystem toolkit, which can be found at *http://dms.dartmouth.edu/cms/*

Look

These tools allow you to visualize environments and activities that form the innovation challenge. They facilitate seeing the whole system in action including the dynamic interactions of actors in the system.

Tool 3: photo survey

Description
A photo survey is a scripted visual portrayal of the people, process, and tools used in the experience under exploration.

Use
1. Create a shooting script
2. Perform the photo shoot
3. Display photos as montage
4. Annotate photos

A shooting script defines the specific activities, peoples, and materials that will be photographed during the photo shoot.

Photos are printed and displayed on a montage board in the layout of the process observed.

The photographer annotates appropriate photos with observations, comments, and ideas for innovating.

Tool 4: activity mapping (spaghetti diagram)

Description
Virtually all service and many product innovations require movement. To better understand how movement/activity is occurring in the existing process or using the existing product, it is highly valuable to track and map the movements of actors within the setting (Figure 3.4).

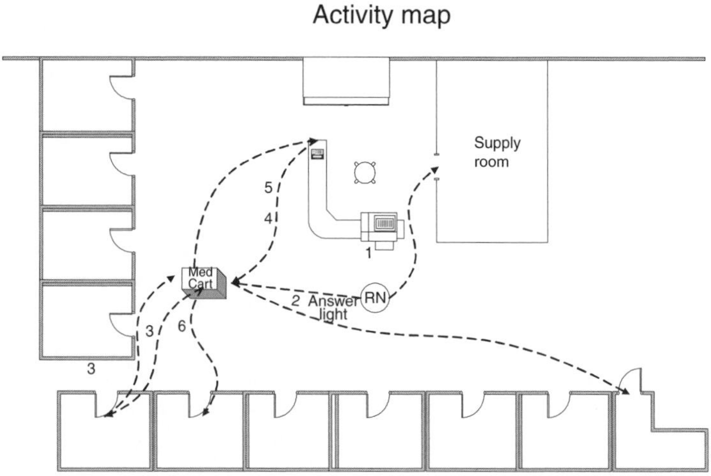

Activity map

Figure 3.4 Spaghetti diagram.

Use

1. Start with drawing the physical layout of the setting where the innovation challenge resides, e.g., hospital unit, emergency department, and clinical office
2. Define all the usual actors and assign a unique symbol for each
3. For a given process, draw lines (and number) for movements of actor
4. Review with your innovation team to determine where opportunities for streamlining and innovation might occur (and place within the diagram)

Resources

The UK National Health Services Institute for Innovation and Improvement provides guidance on construction of a spaghetti diagram –*www.nodelaysachiever.nhs.uk/ServiceImprovement/ Tools/IT215_Spaghetti_Diagram.htm*

Appendix A provides a sample template for your activity map.

Tool 5: behavioral mapping/behavioral archeology

Description

Observing and recording the activities of people in the environment of interest can reveal patterns of activities and use of artifacts that can inform the idea generation process. Behavioral mapping is a drawing of how actors in the environment of interest move and act. Behavioral archeology is the recording of the artifacts that people use or encounter, how they are arranged in space, and their use patterns.

Use

1. Arrange with the manager of the environment time and access to record activities
2. Find a location in the environment where you will be least obstructive
3. Record the people and roles who are active
4. Draw a rough sketch of the physical environment
5. Map the movements of the people during a given period of time (e.g., 1 hour)
6. Record what physical objects that the people use or interact with
7. Bring samples of objects and the behavioral map to the innovation group for discussion of innovation opportunities

Resources

Dr Michael Schiffer, the father of behavioral archeology, has written a seminal text entitled *Behavioral Archeology* that describes useful methods.

Appendix B provides a sample behavioral archeology form.

Tool 6: behavior sampling

Description

Self-recorded samples of behaviors can be illuminating of the innovation topic, serving as a method for capturing the experience, activities, and artifacts of the users in the environment.

Use

1. Select a representative group of individuals in the environment of interest
2. Provide each a pager or cell phone
3. Provide each a recording note (pocket size)
4. Periodically page or call individual

5. Each individual when paged or called records what they are doing, what they are using, with whom they are interacting, and
how they are feeling

Tool 7: process mapping

Description
Process mapping is the visual representation of the steps and activities for a specific process (e.g., a patient visit, and an emergency
department triage event). Process maps can be simple or complex
depending on the information recorded. For instance, beyond the
steps involved, the time taken, the accuracy and completeness of
the activity, the artifacts used including the information exchanged
may be recorded (Figure 3.5).

Use
1. Identify the process to study
2. Define the start and end points
3. Identify all the participants in the process
4. Ask the participants as a group to define all the steps in the process (useful to record on sticky notes so that they can be moved
   around a flipchart)
5. Ask the group to order the steps and identify what is occurring
   at each step (activities, materials, information exchange, etc.)
6. Ask for consensus on the final map (current state map)
7. Ask for suggestions for improvements in the process (future state
   map)
   Some key considerations are (a) write down the objectives of the
process before mapping, (b) keep the process to five to eight steps,
and (c) identify decision points and activity loops.

Resources
The American Society for Quality has a variety of quality tools that
are helpful. Among them is a flowchart tool found at ***www.asq.
org/learn-about-quality/process-analysis-tools/overview/flowchart.
html*** Another excellent resource is the Quality ToolBook found
at ***syque.com/quality_tools/toolbook/toolbook.htm*** HealthInsight,
the Quality Improvement Organization for Utah, provides a free
process mapping software (Workflow 1.0) that allows simple to

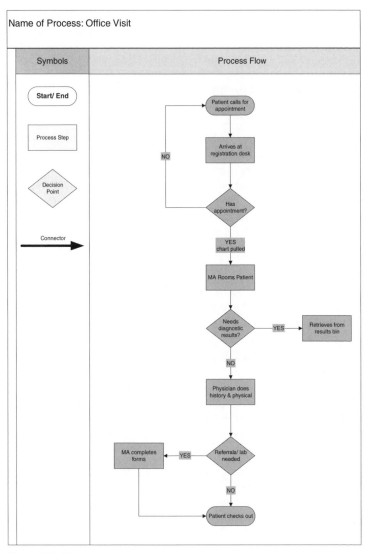

Figure 3.5 Process map.

complex mapping of healthcare processes. It enables tagging of process steps that can be automated or streamlined; see *www. healthinsight.org/hcp/doqit/workflow.html.*

Appendix C provides a blank process map to help guide your mapping exploration of the innovation challenge.

Ask

One of the best ways to get into the mind of the user and understand the experience embodied in the innovation challenge is to inquire. Chapter 2 described an approach to "Discovery Interviews" that is also applicable to deep dive explorations as well.

Tool 8: 5 whys

Description
Under many opportunities for innovation lie unrecognized connections and assumptions. The five whys have been used in quality improvement efforts to reach the heart of the problem. It is an easy and often surprising way to identify the real influences on a process, and opens up new opportunity for innovation.

Use
1. State the innovation challenge
2. Ask why this is a challenge
3. For each subsequent answer or hypothesis, ask why again
4. Record each answer
5. Repeat for at least five times

Example
The example given in Table 3.1 highlights that there are often hidden issues within the innovation challenge. In the overcrowded

Table 3.1 Five whys example

Why	Response
Why is the emergency department always overcrowded?	Emergency department beds are always full.
Why are the emergency department beds always full?	There are delays in opening beds on the floors.
Why are there delays in floor beds?	Patients are not discharged in a timely fashion.
Why are patients not discharged in a timely fashion?	Discharge planner does not see patient till day of discharge.
Why do discharge planners not see patients till day of discharge?	Order for discharge planning variably written by physician on the last day.

emergency department example, the constraint in the system is the process of discharge planning. Until that problem is fixed, other solutions, while they may improve emergency department crowding, will only backlog patients behind the discharge.

Tool 9: KAP surveys

Description
KAP surveys are methods to collect a range of data from providers, patients, and others about the innovation challenge. Knowledge refers to what the respondent knows about a disease, a care strategy, a care institution, or a provider. KAP surveys are also valuable as premarketing assessments to determine viability of a new product or service.

Use
1. Design the survey
2. Identify the target audience
3. Conduct the survey
4. Perform the analysis
5. Present to the innovation team

Example
Patient survey of chest pain behaviors is given in Table 3.2.

Resource
The American Society for Quality offers guidance on use of surveys to collect data for improvement that can be found

Table 3.2 KAP survey example

Knowledge
1. Have you heard of the acute coronary syndrome?
2. What are the symptoms that indicate you should call 911?

Attitude
3. Do you prefer medications or surgery for blocked blood vessels in your heart?
4. How likely are you to tell your doctor about your symptoms?

Practice
5. What is the first thing you do when you get chest pain?
6. Do you miss taking your medications?

at *www.asq.org/learn-about-quality/data-collection-analysis-tools/ overview/survey.html*

Appendix D provides a sample customer survey template.

Tool 10: unfocus groups

Description

Unfocus groups, unlike focus groups that are composed of "typical users," are assemblies of individuals with unique perspectives and passion about the innovation challenge. For instance, IDEO was designing a new fashion sandal and put together a group comprised by an artist, a foot-fetishist, a podiatrist, and others. The goal of an unfocus group is to not only to exchange perspectives, but also to allow them to interact with a range of materials and put together mock-ups or prototypes. Unfocus groups can also use informance (described below) to more vividly describe their experiences with the innovation challenge topic.

Use

1. Identify types of individuals who might give the broadest and interesting range of perspectives on the innovation topic
2. Organize a group session
3. Ask participants to share their experiences with the innovation topic
4. Solicit ideas for innovation
5. Provide them materials such as drawing paper and Styrofoam/cardboard, and ask them to craft crude prototypes of their ideas and/or
6. Ask them to act out (informance) their ideas
7. Elicit feedback from the rest of the group

Tool 11: mind mapping

Description

Mind maps are a technique developed by Anthony Buzan, PhD, as a visual way of exploring problems. It is useful for both problem identification and problem solution. Mind maps are built on the foundation of mental association, and the incredible fact that our minds are considerably more facile in dealing with images than words. Like the five whys, Mind Maps are a fast and easy way to dig into the underlying assumptions and experiences related to the innovation challenge.

Use

1. Draw a circle in the center of your paper, with the innovation challenge inside
2. As associations come to mind about the innovation challenge, draw them as radiant branches from the core or from the new branch as subbranches (see example in Figure 3.6)
3. Use lots of color and images
4. Have fun
5. Share your mind maps with your innovation team and explain the branches to them

Resources

A good place to start is Buzan's book, *The Mind Map Book.*[2] The Innovation Network offers an online eight-step outline of how to create and use mind maps. It can be found at ***http://www.mind-mapping.co.uk/make-mind-map.htm***. There are also a number of mind-mapping software such as MindMapper, Visual Mind, and Mindjet. FreeMind is a free software application that can be downloaded from ***freemind.sourceforge.net/wiki/index.php/Main_Page***.

Appendix E provides a mind-mapping template.

Try

One of the most powerful tools for exploring an innovation challenge is to try out or model existing and potential experiences. Chapter 5 provides suggestions for building models of prototyping, but it is never too early to start putting models together. Tim Brown from IDEO describes this as "prototyping as thinking."

Tool 12: informance

Description

Actions speak louder than words. Informance is the acting out of scenarios related to the innovation topic. They can be performed by the innovation team (especially after the observation period) or an unfocus group. The benefit is that a shared understanding of the user experience is developed.

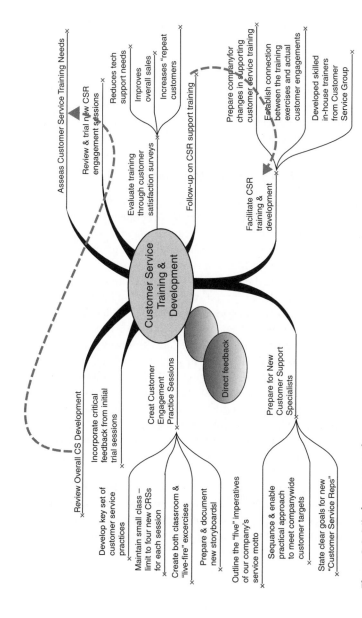

Figure 3.6 Mind map example.

Use
1. Define the set of actors (innovation group, unfocus group, others)
2. Define a set of scenarios relevant to the innovation topic
3. Ask the actors to act out the experience
4. Solicit clarifications from the actors regarding activities, materials, and experience encountered

Resource
IDEO has produced a guide for conducting role explorations through informance and bodystorming. See Appendix F for guidance on creating a role-playing process as part of the deep dive into your innovation challenge.

An innovation story continued

The innovation team undertook a deep dive to better understand hospital discharges and readmissions at Greenfield Health Systems. During one week, the team observed and mapped ten consecutive discharges from five units at the hospital. They mapped each step that was observed from the time that the discharge order was written to the time that the patient was admitted to another facility, such as a nursing home or returned home, and resumed caring for themselves. In this process, they also did in-depth interviews of patients being discharged from the hospital, resuming care at home, and being readmitted to hospital with an unexpected complication. The team spent a day in the home of ten patients just discharged from hospital, observing and photographing resuming of home-based care. In addition, the team drew activity maps of nursing unit discharge activities. In the innovation team room, as data was gathered, it was posted on a project wall as a montage that included photos that were annotated, summaries of interviews with direct quotes, maps of process and activities, and summaries of the literature from the "defining challenge" stage. On the day that information gathering was completed, the team assembled and discussed what was found, distilling out major themes. Key themes were lack of information on self-care and follow-up, confusion about restarting medications, and the resulting lack of continuity of care.

Appendix A: activity/spaghetti diagram

Venue Name

Actors				
Actor 1	Actor 2	Actor 3	Actor 4	

Layout

Appendix B: behavioral archeology form

Behavioral Archeology

Name of Venue: _____

Instructions: Record specific artifacts in the venue, who/how they are used, ideas for innovation

Table 3.3 Behavioral archeology template

Artifacts	Who Uses/ How Used	Innovation Opportunity

Appendix C: process mapping form

Name of Process Venue:	
Symbols	**Process Flow**
Start/ End	
Process Step	
Decision Point	
Connector ➤	

Appendix D: customer survey template
Customer Interview Summary

Name of Venue: _____

Instructions: explain that you are members of an innovation team from [your organization] learning about innovation and would like to ask them a few questions about their experience at this venue.

Table 3.4 Customer survey template

Question	Responses
Q1. How often do you come here?	
Q2. What do you like most about this place?	
Q3. What could they improve?	
Q4. What do they not offer now that you think would make this a better place?	

Appendix E: mind map process

Your Mind Map of Innovation Topic

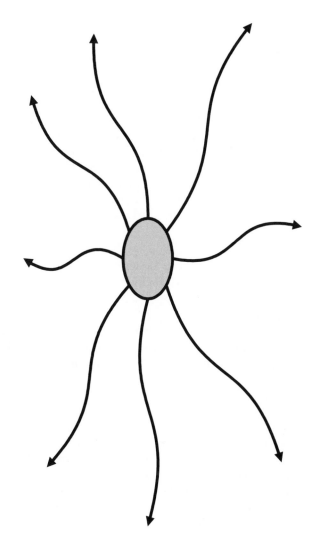
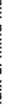

Appendix F: role-playing process

Take it to the Next Stage:
The Roles of Role Playing in the Design
Process

Kristian T. Simsarian
IDEO – San Francisco Pier 28 Annex, The Embarcadero,
San Francisco, CA 94105 415-615-5051, ksimsarian@ideo.com

ABSTRACT
Using role play at every stage of the design process has been a vital tool for IDEO in working with clients and users. With the dual properties of bringing participants into the moment and making shared activities physical rather than just mental, role playing techniques make the process more experiential and creatively generative. Role playing is complementary to traditional design techniques providing additional team dynamics and insights that bring the process and designs to another level. This paper describes how we have used role-playing in our design process and how it can be integrated into any HCI project.

Keywords
Bodystorming, participatory design, improve, role playing, rapid prototyping, scenarios, collaborative design.

INTRODUCTION
In today's design projects, whiteboards, talking heads and PowerPoint slides are not enough. IDEO has developed experiential role-playing techniques that bring insights and communication to a new level.

IDEO's design practice has grown from engineering and industrial design to include innovative service, environment, and organizational design. Projects often include new-to-the-world systemic and strategic brand issues as well as interactive systems that are highly nuanced and difficult to articulate verbally. Because such projects are close to client's core goals, we often work shoulder-to-shoulder with multi-disciplinary stakeholders from all levels including executives. With strategic design briefs of "what could be" and participants with different backgrounds and goals, simply being in the room together and capturing ideas in written form often leaves participants with unresolved individual issues, differing mental conceptions, and unresolved details. Role playing can work to bring it all together.

Building on previously described work on experiential methods [2], participatory design work with children [1] and bodystorming [3] the role playing techniques described in this paper not only overcome many of the group issues but also make the process fun and exciting.

The Role Playing Difference

What is role playing? Role playing is the practice of group physical and spatial pretend where individuals deliberately assume a character role in a constructed scene with, or without, props. The key differentiating aspects of role playing are: 1) Being "in the moment" - an individual and group state that enables vivid and focused exploration of the situations and 2) Physicalization - using the entire body to explore generation of ideas that takes "brainstorming" to "bodystorming." This sort of role playing is similar to the practice of improve theater [4]. These two factors can be seen as defining qualities and goals for the practice. Being in the moment and physicalization provide the basis for role playing's greatest benefits:

- Maintaining group focus on the activities at hand;
- Bringing teams onto the "same page" through a shared vivid experience that involves
- participant's muscle memory;
- Deferring judgment while building on other's ideas;
- Building deeper understanding grounded in context;
- The ability to viscerally explore possibilities that may not be readily available in the world.

PHASED ROLE PLAYING

IDEO projects often proceed in phases. Different types of role play are relevant to these different phases. The phases occur in the sequence: Understand, Observe, Visualize, Evaluate, Refine and Implement. Throughout many techniques are employed such as observation, storyboarding, user studies, prototyping, and workshops. While many of these techniques are powerful, few focus on intergroup communication and bringing about rapid group understanding. Role play can be used in all phases of the design process from Understand through to final concept Implementation and transfer

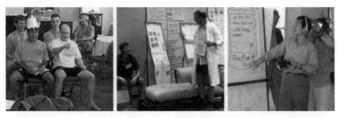

Figure 3.7 Figure 10: From left to right: Working with a financial services company to design new travel services, working with the NIH to envision optimal research collaboration strategies, working with a hardware manufacturer to explore new PDA services.

to the client and customer. Role playing has unique and specific usefulness for each phase of the design process:

- **Understand – "Where to look"** Issue discovery and identification that grounds the team. Performing walk-throughs to uncover issues and nuances that inform early work and identify the questions to ask.
- **Observation: "Re-creations"** Sharing understandings from the field, recreating observed situations or creating extrapolations based on an understanding of the observations.
- **Visualization: "Bodystorming"** Doing generative work: exploring contexts to develop new ideas and uses. This work is often informed by the opportunity themes that emerge from observation.
- **Evaluation & Refinement: "Debugging"** Building scenarios of use, discovering hidden nuances and tuning. Working out, and working through, details of possible scenarios before delivery or implementation.
- **Implementation: "Informance" (Informative Performance)** The practice of creating physical performances to communicate developed ideas, issues, and scenarios to an audience. Informances might also be used in any design phase to convey current ideas and issues in a rich way.

DOING IT
These different aspects of role play can be used throughout the design process and become part of the way the team works. Two techniques are particularly well suited for use together: **Bodystorming** and **Informance**. We have found that these can be used in a half

or full day structured workshop even with complete beginners. The output is a rich experience and a set of performed scenarios on video. Such a workshop might have 8-20 participants broken out into teams of 3-5 persons with the given sample agenda.

Time	Sample Agenda
0:00	Field Observation (or "what we know" session) to ground the group in understanding the design problem and opportunities
1:30	Brainstorm using the opportunities to generate as many ideas as possible by creating a space where anything is possible
2:30	Post-it™ vote on brainstorm ideas, e.g. "easiest" and "greatest impact" creating a set of selected ideas.
3:00	Break into teams, where each group takes one of the selected ideas. These groups detail the ideas by exploring it through bodystorming and use the best elements and ideas to develop a scenario.
4:00	Reconvene groups for Informance – each team presents their scenario - which is videoed. The videos may be reviewed to capture issues.

This workshop format has been used in both early and mid-stage projects. It is equally well suited to kick-off meetings and when exploring design details. We regularly use these techniques in both our design projects and in our IDEO U courses where we teach clients rapid design and innovation techniques. These clients have included product and service companies such as Fujitsu, American Express, Reuters, Lilly, P&G, United Media, DePaul Hospital as well as government entities such as the FBI, the IRS and the NIH.

Role Playing Tips

We find that videotaping not only provides documentation, but also sharpens the performances. Roles can be anything, persons, emotions, things; it can help to instruct that "each scenario will have at least one new role and one non-human role." IDEO's standard brainstorming rules are equally relevant to role playing: defer judgment, encourage wild ideas, build on the ideas of others, stay focused on the topic, and one conversation at a time. The notion of breakout teams introduces both deadlines and aspects of team competition that help to focus participants on the goals. In addition to reviewing basic workshop skills, facilitators may also wish to explore improvisation exercises and warm-ups [4]. An ample and diverse supply of costumes and props helps to set the stage for creative fun.

ACKNOWLEDGMENTS

Thanks to the creative people both at IDEO and the clients we work with for providing many opportunities and much support and fun while exploring and refining these ideas.

CHI 2003, April 5–10, 2003, Ft. Lauderdale, Florida, USA.

REFERENCES

1. Benford, S. *et al*, Designing Storytelling Technologies to Encourage Collaboration Between Young Children, in *Proceedings of CHI'00*, (The Hague, 2000), ACM Press, 556–563.
2. Buchenau, M. and Fulton Suri, J., Experience Prototyping in *Proceedings on Designing Interactive Systems (NY, NY 2000), ACM Press*, 424–433.
3. Burns, C. *et al*, Actors, Hairdos & Videotape – Informance Design, in *Proceedings of CHI'94*, (Boston, MA 1994), ACM Press, 119–120.
4. Johnstone, K., *Impro for Storytellers*, Routledge 1999.

References

1. Brown T. "Strategy by Design." Fast Company, June 2005, pp. 2–5.
2. Buzan T, Buzan B. *The Mind Map Book*, Penguin Books, New York, 1993.

CHAPTER 4
Generating innovative ideas

The heart of innovation is generating and testing of new ideas. Generating new ideas requires the innovator to think differently—to move beyond the usual way of thinking or seeing the world. There are over 200 published methods for creative idea generation; as Paul Plsek[1] has said, "anything that helps us pay attention in a different way, escape our current mental patterns, and maintain movement in our thoughts" aid the process of generating innovative ideas. All methods for creating new ideas fall into one or more of these three categories.

> **The world we have made as a result of the level of thinking we have done thus far creates problems we cannot solve at the same level of thinking at which we created them.**
>
> Albert Einstein

Attention –Escape–Movement

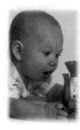 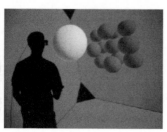 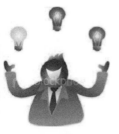

| Attention | Escape | Movement |

Innovation in Action: A practical guide for healthcare teams, 1st edition.
By D. Scott Endsley. © 2010 Blackwell Publishing.

To be an effective and creative innovator means that you must learn to use both sides of your brain. Left-brain skills enable you to see deeper logical connections and effectively challenge your working assumptions. The TRIZ (Theory of Inventive Problem Solving) tools described below are a good example of left-brain idea generating tools. Right-brain skills enable you to break out of engrained assumptions and modes of thinking/behaving. Lateral thinking tools are great right-brain tools. Great innovators practice constantly using both sides of the brain, and look for ways of bringing the two together. They exercise both sides of their brains, and have great corpus callosums!

Where can you start? The DirectedCreativity Web site provides a number of tools and strategies for creative thinking (*www.directedcreativity.com*). Mindtools is another site with excellent resource (*www.mindtools.com*). CreatingMinds offers an electronic creativity toolbox (*www.creatingminds.org*). The Creativity and Innovation, Science and Technology Web site is another wonderful resource with creativity tools (*www.mycoted.com/Category:Creativity_Techniques*). Final is Michael Michalko's book, *ThinkerToys*,[2] which is also available by subscription on his Web site *www.thinkertoys.biz*.

As you explore and develop your skills as a creative idea generator and innovator, it is useful to have some basic "rules of thumb" in your work. My favorites are Paul Plsek's[3] eight heuristics for innovative thinking:

1. Make a habit to purposefully pause and notice things
2. Focus your creative energies on just a few topics that you care about
3. Avoid being too narrow in how you define your topic
4. Try to come up with original and useful ideas by making novel associations among what you already know
5. When you need creative ideas remember 'attention–escape–movement'
6. Pause and carefully examine ideas that make you laugh the first time
7. Recognize that your streams of thought and patterns of judgment are not inherently right or wrong
8. Make a deliberate effort to harvest, develop, and implement at least a few of the ideas you generate

DirectedCreativity model

A very useful model that describes the creative process for healthcare innovation has been proposed by Paul Plsek, a leading thinker about healthcare innovation. His model called *DirectedCreativity*[TM4] (Figure 4.1) has four phases, which are consistent with the innovation model described in Chapter 1. It begins with observation of the things, interactions, and processes contained in our innovation challenge and evaluated with considered analysis. These form the floor on which the imagination can dance and generate new ideas through lateral thinking and concept association, which are in turn prioritized and harvested to find the most viable for further prototyping or development. These prototyped ideas are put to the test and evaluated for their viability in the real world. Plsek identifies tools for each of these four phases, which include:

- Preparation
- Imagination
- Development
- Action

There are two phases of idea generation. The first phase is dedicated to finding a wide array of ideas through techniques that focus attention, allow us to escape usual patterns of thinking and belief, and move our thinking. The second phase then harvests

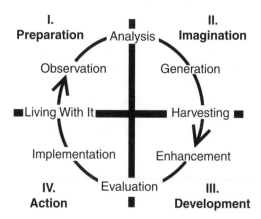

Figure 4.1 DirectedCreativity model. (Reproduced with permission from Paul E., Plsek & Associates, Inc. *www.directedcreativity.com*.)

Brainstorming Solutions for Nurse Knowledge Exchange. Kaiser Permanente and its innovation consultancy brought together multidisciplinary teams from four regions to design solutions for better knowledge exchange during shift change (described in Chapter 3). These teams included frontline nurses, physicians, pharmacists, bed managers, information technology specialists, and national experts. Deep dive findings from the four sites were presented to the innovation teams. A 2-hour brainstorming session was held, with over 100 ideas generated. A nominal group process narrowed down the potential ideas to 4, with the greatest merit including staggered shift changes, care boards, shift preparation, bedside rounds. These were rapidly prototyped and bodystormed, with additional refinements to the ideas.

these ideas, narrowing down the ideas that have the greatest promise of working, and selecting a small set of ideas to begin prototyping.

Finding new ideas

Tool 1: treasure chest

Description
Some of the best ideas for innovative services and products are derivative of ideas of others. A treasure chest is a manifestation of Plsek's first heuristic to purposefully notice things. It is a way of unleashing your thought process by collecting examples of innovative design that can serve to stimulate your thinking about your design (Figure 4.2).

Use
1. Stay attentive to ideas, things and materials, and processes that strike you as surprising; these can come from anywhere: a toy store, hardware store, an airport check-in, and a hotel encounter
2. Collect them and store them in a "treasure chest" – a box or tool cabinet or anything that is able to hold a wide variety of objects. A key aspect of the "treasure chest" is the ability to separate things of different nature such as photographs and drawings,

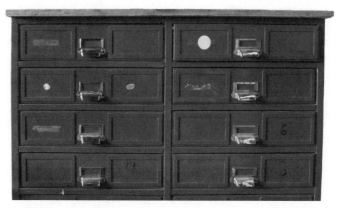

Figure 4.2 Treasure chest.

interesting materials, and creatively designed objects. A potential treasure chest is a used medication cart from a hospital unit

3. If unable to purchase or obtain them (e.g., a creative use of materials on a bridge), draw or photograph them
4. During unfocus groups or informance or other idea-generating activities, bring out samples from the treasure chest to stimulate thinking

Tool 2: brainstorming

Description
There is a Japanese proverb that says "none of us are as smart as all of us." Generating ideas as a collective exercise is one of the best ways to generate a lot of ideas out of which may come a great idea (or two). Brainstorming involves assembling your interdisciplinary innovation team, providing them an innovation challenge and allowing them enough time, tools, and enthusiasm to generate and prioritize a number of good ideas. It is something that needs to be a habit and practiced often. IDEO has found that a good brainstormer can generate over 100 ideas in an hour. They have identified "seven secrets for better brainstorming,"[5] which include:

1. *Sharpen the focus.* Start with a crisp but simple innovation challenge statement that is high level enough not to drive the group toward predetermine solutions
2. *Playful rules.* IDEO has created rules such as "defer judgement, go for quantity, encourage wild ideas, be visual, build on the ideas of others," and stay away from critique or debate

3. *Number your ideas.* It's a great way to monitor flow of ideas and to move back and forth between ideas. It also allows easier affinity grouping and prioritization
4. *Build and jump.* A facilitator encourages participants to take someone else's idea and build off of it or switch gears. This is analogous to building a mind map through associations and branches
5. *Space remembers.* Capture ideas so that everyone can see and build upon. Don't be afraid of covering the walls. Allow participants to wander around the room
6. *Stretch your mental muscles.* Try a mental warm-up before you get started, especially when the group hasn't worked together before or hasn't work together for a while. This exercise can come in several types: brief warm-ups with word or mind games (see ***www.mycoted.com/Category:Puzzles*** for examples of mind games) or prework prior to the brainstormer such as a Google or library search on the innovation topic
7. *Get physical.* Use a variety of visual techniques to depict and stimulate ideas such as sketches, stick figures, diagrams, and maps (including mind maps). It is also a good time to bring in innovative objects from your "treasure chest." It is also a time to start prototyping. Have simple construction materials available to put together scale models. Informance is also helpful in brainstorming to act out an idea

Good brainstorming brings together the best of left and right brain skills. It is an exercise that encompasses both playfulness and discipline. Monitor how the session is going and don't be afraid of making adjustments as a facilitator. One good benchmark is the degree of playfulness and laughter in the group. If you don't hear laughter, the ideas that are being generated probably aren't wild enough. Use some of the lateral thinking skills to get the group off the beaten track.

Use

1. Assemble a group of participants (five to ten) drawn from inside and outside the innovation team. Consider "seeding" the group with a topic expert
2. Set aside an hour (don't go longer) and arrange a comfortable space
3. Provide food, toys, and prototyping materials
4. Facilitator conducts a warm-up exercise (optional)
5. Facilitator presents the innovation challenge

6. Participants offer ideas written down by the facilitator on flipcharts, walls, etc. Avoid "going around the table" solicitations
7. Use affinity grouping to cluster ideas into the "big ideas"
8. Use multivoting to select the best ideas to start prototyping and testing

Resources
There are numerous resources to help you get started in gaining mastery of brainstorming. The *Complete Guide to Managing Traditional Brainstorming Events* is a useful resource (***www.jpb.com/creative/ brainstorming.pdf***). The Institute for Healthcare Improvement has a toolsheet on Brainstorming, Affinity Grouping and Multivoting available at ***www.ihi.org/IHI/Topics/Improvement/Improvement Methods/Tools/Brainstorming+Affinity+Grouping+Multivoting.htm***. A variety of brainstorming tools and software are available at ***www.innovationtools.com***.

Tool 3: bodystorming

Description
While brainstorming focuses on ideas and sometimes prototypes, bodystorming focuses on using action to understand and create new processes, services, or products. It involves defining a scenario and acting it out based on what is understood about the innovation challenge (Figure 4.3).

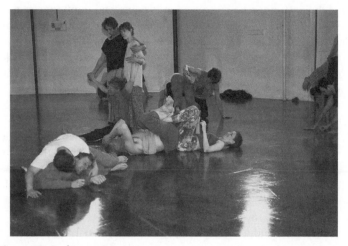

Figure 4.3 Bodystorming.

Use
1. Based on information from the innovation assessment step (Chapter 3), define one or more scenarios that represent the innovation challenge
2. Have your innovation team select actors
3. Actors play out the scenario based on what they know
4. Get feedback and ideas from the innovation team on new variations in the scenario and act them out
5. Repeat this cycle until enough ideas are generated

It is helpful to video the scenarios as they are acted out and review them with the innovation team.

Tool 4: lateral thinking

Description
Much as a stream follows a well-worn bed, our thinking tends to follow the paths of previous thinking, often in rote and mechanical ways. The challenge for innovators is to discover untread paths in thinking that leads to different perspectives that enlighten innovation efforts. Dr Edward deBono, a renown English psychologist, first proposed that truly creative thinking derives from moving laterally rather than vertically in thinking. He devised a series of strategies to help the mind stop digging the hole in the same place but to look for other places to dig. Four are highlighted here: *Po statements, analogies, the reversal method,* and *concept fans.*

Use
1. *Po statements.* These are outrageous statements meant to provoke mental movement. The provocative statement is signaled by introducing it with the work "Po." For example, "Po, doctors change their schedules to meet the needs of their patients" or "Po, patients only pay if they are happy with the care received"
2. *Analogies.* These are adapted ideas and strategies from other settings. For instance, bar coding in healthcare is an adaptation of bar coding in the mercantile industry. How might the hotel industry's method for tracking customers' preference be used in healthcare?
3. *Reversal method.* This strategy explicitly turns assumptions on their heads. It is a provocative strategy intended to shift thinking. For instance, if the usual is that physicians write prescriptions for patients, the reversal statement might be "the patient writes

Current process   Concept   Alternatives

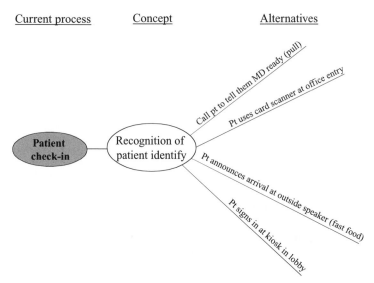

Figure 4.4 Concept fan.

prescriptions for physicians or simply the patient writes prescriptions." What would happen if this reversed situation were to occur? Are there benefits or harms? What could be done to enable the reversed situation without causing harm?

4. *Concept fans.* This is a high-level process map (up to five or six steps) that links the underlying concepts or assumptions for each step, and then provides alternatives to the current concept. See Figure 4.4 for an example. It is a wonderful tool to explore possible solutions that emanate from a central concept. An excellent guide to concept fan construction can be found at ***www.mindtools.com/pages/article/newCT_06.htm***

   Lateral thinking methods can be used as stand-alone tools to help in idea generation or can be integrated into other idea generation activities such as unfocus groups and brainstorming. Like other creativity skills, lateral thinking takes frequent practice to make them effective.

Resources

Edward de Bono's book *Lateral Thinking*[6] is the starting point for anyone interested in lateral thinking methodologies. His Web site is also very useful (***www.debonogroup.com***). There is also a software application developed by the deBono group, *DeBono 24 × 7*, that provides Web-based assistance in applying lateral thinking methods to your innovation challenge. It is available at ***www. debonogroup.com/software.htm*** with ***www.debonogroup.com***. Paul Plsek[1] has described several of deBono's methods as applied in healthcare.

Tool 5: TRIZ

Description

The Theory of Inventive Problem Solving (TRIZ for short) was formulated by a Russian scientist Genrich Altshuller in the 1940s. He discovered that many inventions were successful because they resolved a physical contradiction. For instance, how do you simultaneously improve speed *and* strength of a vehicle (such as an airplane)? He identified 40 principles for design that are applied singly or in multiples to resolve a contradiction inhibiting the design. In addition, 39 material features (e.g., weight and durability,) have been delineated which characterize the contradiction (e.g., speed vs strength). A contradiction matrix has been developed that identifies which of the 40 principles applies to the pair of contradictory material features (see ***www.triz40.com***) (Figure 4.5).

Use

1. Define the specific innovation challenge
2. Restate the challenge in general, higher level terms

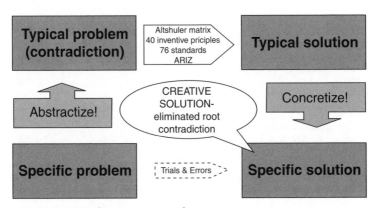

Figure 4.5 TRIZ idea generation path.

3. Identify what are the contradictions contained in the challenge
4. Identify which of the 40 principles would resolve the contradiction
5. Define the solution produced by resolution of the contradiction
6. Redefine the solution in specific terms for the innovation challenge

Resources

Altschuler's seminal work *And Suddenly the Inventor Appeared*[7] provides a comprehensive overview of the TRIZ methodology and many examples from industry. TRIZ40 provides a free online contradiction matrix available at ***www.triz40.com***.

Tool 6: stepping stones

Description

This tool is drawn from the *Thinking Differently* guide produced by the UK Institution for Innovation and Improvement (which is available at ***www.institute.nhs.uk/building_capability/new_model_ for_transforming_the_nhs/thinking_differently_guide.html***). This tool acts as a catalyst for innovation teams to leap from a seemingly wild idea to those that might be buildable ideas. Starting with outrageous starting points and assumptions frees the mind from having to honor logic (if only for the moment). This allows flights of ideas and challenging of assumptions that might lead to useful ideas for further prototyping and development (Figure 4.6).

Example:
Innovation Challenge: Organization doesn't see value of innovation in daily work

Outrageous Idea: All employees' job descriptions require 20% minimum time innovating their work

Underlying concepts:
• Innovation produces value
• All employees are innovators
• Innovation skills are considered organization competencies
• All work is considered candidate for innovation

Change ideas:
• Explicitly defining business case for innovation
• Integrating innovation goals into employee performance evaluation
• Employee innovation training program

Figure 4.6 Stepping stone example.

Use

1. State your innovation challenge
2. Propose an outrageous solution irrespective of its practicality. In fact, the less practical but provocative, the better
3. List all the underlying concepts or assumptions in the idea
4. Connect how these concepts or assumptions be applied in the workplace to the innovation challenge at hand

Resource

The NHS's *Thinking Differently* guide has a variety of idea-generating tools useful for healthcare organizations. It can be found at *www.institute.nhs.uk/building_capability/new_model_for_transforming_the_nhs/thinking_differently_guide.html*.

Tool 7: that's impossible

Description

This tool is also derived from the *Thinking Differently* guide produced by the UK Institution for Innovation and Improvement.[8] This tool challenges the innovator to consider possibilities beyond the accepted norm. Remember though that yesterday's impossibilities are today's realities. For instance, at the beginning of the twentieth century, it was considered impossible that man would fly. Now flying is the preferred way of traveling (Figure 4.7).

Use

1. Create a list of things that are thought to be impossible today
2. Brainstorm how the impossible could become possible

Example:
That's impossible: Managing a heart attack in the patient's home

What makes it possible
- Remote EKG monitoring
- Physician "control tower"
- "Intelligent" IV pumps
- Interactive digital pictures

Figure 4.7 That's impossible example.

Resource
NHS's *Thinking Differently* guide.

Tool 8: seeing through others eyes

Description
This tool is also derived from the *Thinking Differently* guide produced by the UK Institution for Innovation and Improvement.[8] This tool fits closely with experience-based design approaches by bring the perspectives and ideas of non-healthcare people into consideration.

Use
1. State the innovation challenge
2. Select a non-healthcare viewpoint such as that of a child, baker, accountant, mother, airline pilot, research scientist, politician, or some other role
3. Ask how this viewpoint might see the innovation challenge:
   - What would be important to them
   - What expertise would they apply to the challenge
   - What approaches would they take to the challenge

Resource
NHS's *Thinking Differently* guide. An alternative group model of this is the unfocus group.

Harvesting ideas

Once you have generated a list of ideas that range from the slightly different to the wildly odd, the innovator needs to sort out those with the greatest potential for the development in the prototyping phase. The three tools described below assist the innovation team in evaluating the value of ideas.

Tool 9: multivoting

Description
This technique allows each member of the innovation team to express his or her preference for specific ideas. By allowing members to cast multiple votes for different ideas, a small set of ideas can be rapidly culled.

Use
1. Ask the team to review the ideas generated and group them based on similarity. This is called affinity grouping
2. Discuss the most appropriate descriptive label for each group
3. Provide three to five colored dots (sticky dots on a sheet work well) to each member and ask them to stick them next to the ideas they think are the best. They may use one dot for different ideas or may put more than one dot on an idea
4. When complete, count the dots and identify five to seven ideas that got the most votes
5. Use the Six Hats and Depth of Innovation tools described below

Resources
The American Society for Quality offers instruction on how to conduct a multivoting session (***www.asq.org/learn-about-quality/ decision-making-tools/overview/mutivoting.html***). The Institute for Healthcare Improvement also offers a toolsheet for brainstorming, affinity grouping, and multivoting, which can be found at ***www.ihi.org/IHI/Topics/Improvement/ImprovementMethods/Tools/ Brainstorming+Affinity+Grouping+Multivoting.htm***.

Tool 10: depth of innovation tool

Description
This tool developed by Paul Plsek asks the innovation team to rate a particular idea on its innovativeness. The rating scale has six gradations, from usual thinking to original thinking (Table 4.1).

Use
1. Record the ideas culled during the multivoting process on the form provided in Appendix A
2. Ask each member to rate the innovativeness on the scale of 1 to 6
3. Sum the scores for each idea
4. Identify the highest scoring idea

Resource
Appendix A provides a description and the Depth of Innovation Scale developed by Paul Plsek.

Table 4.1 Depth of innovation rating

Usual thinking	This idea is the typical approach to the topic at hand. It is the way that most people in our industry (here, healthcare) handle it. Most similar teams, groups, departments, or organizations in our industry (healthcare) are already doing something very similar to this
Potential better practice thinking	This idea is an adaptation of ideas that are becoming somewhat common in other organizations in my industry (here, healthcare), but it is still a fairly new idea. Only one-third or fewer similar teams, groups, departments, or organizations in our industry (healthcare) are doing something like this
Clever thinking	This idea is a really clever twist on our existing ways of doing things, it is creative thinking on a small scale
Creative connection thinking	This idea is a creative adaptation of ideas and concepts that are common outside my industry, but rarely used within my industry (here, ideas that are common outside healthcare, but not common within healthcare)
Paradigm busting thinking	This idea fundamentally challenges current mental models and paradigms in our industry (here, healthcare) in an uncommon way; it is creative thinking on a deeper scale
Original thinking	This idea is really a new concept and is truly amazing; no one has ever thought of anything like this before

Plsek P. *http://www.directedcreativity.com/pages/InnovationScale.pdf*, 2007.

Tool 11: Six Hats Tool

Description

This tool adapted from Edward DeBono provides a way of looking at a candidate idea from different perspectives.[8] DeBono proposes that there are six perspectives from which one might look at an innovation challenge or idea. These include the following.

Use

1. Using the form provided in Appendix B, write the idea at the top
2. For each box, take 4 minutes to "wear the hat" and fill each box with:
   - expected benefits in yellow box
   - anticipated negatives and risks in the black box
   - the data or information that would need to be collected in the white box
   - your gut feelings/emotions in the red box

Table 4.2 Six hats thinking

Hat	Description
Black	A cautious perspective that examines the risks, barriers, and negatives of an idea
Blue	A directive perspective that examines the "big picture" and how the idea is managed
Yellow	A positive perspective that examines the benefits of an idea
Red	An emotion-oriented perspective that examines how an idea "feels" or impacts the emotional state of the user
Green	A creative perspective that examines the idea's originality and differentiation
White	A data-oriented perspective that examines the quality of the information relating to the idea, and how it holds up under analytic scrutiny

3. Based on your gestalt of the four boxes taken together, decide whether the idea is a "go" or a "no-go"

Resources
Appendix B provides a Six Hat Evaluation Tool that allows the user to list benefits, risks, data, and gut feeling about an idea in succession.

An innovation story continued

The Greenfield innovation team invited an expanded group from the hospital, including physicians, discharge planners, home nurses, patients, and families to spend one day generating ideas to change the problems of postdischarge follow-up and continuity. The expanded innovation group was presented the findings from "deep dive" and research including the core themes that emerged from these two activities. They were provided an open forum for a dialogue on the significance of each finding. The morning concluded with a 90-minute brainstorming session on ideas on improving the discharge process. Over 100 ideas were proposed, which were grouped into like themes including information sharing, patient activation and support, and connecting the system together. In the afternoon, the group was divided into three groups to continue work on the ideas in each of these three areas. They developed scenarios and skits, and built mock-ups of tools and facilities. At the end of the afternoon, each subteam presented their scenarios (informance) and mock-ups. The whole group voted by the nominal process on the ideas using the four hats priority tool. The highest ranked ideas included (a) a transition plan sheet for patients, (b) use of the in-room television for customized transition education, (c) provision of a health guide made by Intel for the first week with scheduled daily videoconferences between the patient and the hospital discharge team, and (d) establishment of a discharge clinic and hotline for patients unable to be seen by their ambulatory provider within the first 48–72 hours postdischarge.

Appendix A: Plsek depth of innovation scale

How Creative Is That Idea? Thoughts About Creating A Depth of Innovation Scale

Paul Plsek Version 4 Revised April 6, 2004
(from original dated November 7, 2003)
(used with permission)

Introduction and Issue

In working with healthcare organizations using DirectedCreativity™ techniques, discussion often arises about the degree of creativity or innovative-ness of the ideas generated in a session. These notes explore this issue and propose a practical "depth of innovation" scale that I would like to test in several settings.

Understanding the Creative Process

There is general agreement in the literature that the creative process involves connecting and rearranging knowledge in the mind. When someone suggests that hospitals ought to have drive-through windows for dispensing healthcare services, they are making an *unusual* mental connection between two otherwise familiar things. The drive-through window and the hospital are both familiar things; the creative act is to think of them together.

It is the degree of unusualness in the connection (or, the "distance" of the connection) that is typically what we are talking about when we describe the intuitive notion of degrees of creativity. For example, consider these three ideas about ways to deliver services in a new wing of a hospital. . .

1. *"We could have a registration desk and a waiting area, etc."* Here, the person is making a mental connection between the ways services are delivered in other parts of the hospital and how they might be delivered in the new wing. This requires some level of imagination and insight since the new wing does not yet exist, but the connection is not very original. One could say that there is not much mental distance between the current hospital wings and this new one; they are very similar, nearly identical.

2. *"We could install a drive-through window to do lab sample drop-offs, prescription refills, brief education, influenza shots, etc."* Here, we see a connection between how services are dispensed in a fast-food

restaurant and in a hospital. This requires somewhat more imagination. The mental connection is not so typical; there is a greater mental distance between the fast-food industry and a hospital. Therefore, this idea seems more creative than the one above. However, when you stop and think about it, there are some basic similarities between service delivery in fast food and hospitals. Both embrace the paradigm of the customer coming traveling for access to service, and both envision the service delivery happening in a fixed location that belongs to the producer of the service.

3. *"We could create a mobile specialty clinic that could be rapidly set up in a shopping mall or on an employers' premise, etc."* Here, the person is still making connections to existing concepts; we have no trouble imagining a mobile clinic in that we are familiar with large vans and we know that medical personnel and associated equipment could be transported to other places. However, the connections here are a bit more unusual. Unlike the drive-through window idea where the connection with the fast-food industry immediately comes to mind when someone mentions the idea, it is a bit harder to quickly identify an analogous situation in this instance. Perhaps a bookmobile, or a blood drive, or an insurance salesperson who comes to your home—but it is a bit more of a stretch. The mental distance of the connections is, therefore, greater. It is hard to quantify this "distance," but intuitively we can see that it is greater than it was with either of the other two ideas above. Furthermore, this idea challenges some of the fundamental paradigms about service delivery; something that was not as true about idea number 2 above. Here, we are going to the customer and using a non-fixed asset (we could go further and challenge additional paradigms). The fact that fundamental paradigms have been challenged is also linked to our intuitive notion of "distance." In the end, this third idea is more creative than the two before it.

A Proposed "Depth of Innovation" Scale

Any scale designed to answer the question "How creative is this idea?" must reflect this intuitive notion of the unusualness or distance of the mental connection. To be reliable (i.e., two people using the scale to evaluate the same idea would arrive at close to the same rating) the scale must also provide commonly understood anchor points.

I propose the following scale for evaluating an idea. Select an idea for consideration and choose the statement below that you think *best* describes it:

1. **Usual Thinking.** This idea is the typical approach to the topic at hand. It is the way that most people in our industry (here, healthcare) handle it. Most similar teams, groups, departments, or organizations in our industry (healthcare) are already doing something very similar to this.

2. **Potential Better Practice Thinking.** This idea is an adaptation of ideas that are becoming somewhat common in other organizations in my industry (here, healthcare); but it is still a fairly new idea. Only one-third or fewer similar teams, groups, departments, or organizations in our industry (healthcare) are doing something like this.

3. **Clever Thinking.** This idea is a really clever twist on our existing ways of doing things; it is creative thinking on a small scale.

4. **Creative Connection Thinking.** This idea is a creative adaptation of ideas and concepts that are common outside my industry, but rarely used within my industry (here, ideas that are common outside healthcare, but not common within health care).

5. **Paradigm Busting Thinking.** This idea fundamentally challenges current mental models and paradigms in our industry (here, healthcare) in an uncommon way; it is creative thinking on a deeper scale.

6. **Original Thinking.** This idea is really a new concept and is truly amazing; no one has ever thought of anything like this before!

Returning to the three previous examples...

- The idea of providing registration areas, etc. would score a "1." It is useful, but not particularly creative.
- The idea of the drive-through window would score a "4."
- The idea of a mobile clinic in malls and office buildings would score a "5."

To fill out the list...

- An idea about providing open access appointment scheduling would score a "2" because this idea is becoming a common "best practice" in healthcare. Note that for the original pioneers, this idea would have scored much higher. However, over time, ideas that once were considered creative can become common. This is a well-described phenomenon in the innovation literature.

- An idea about having patients come out to the nursing station on the floor to get their own medications from the nurse at appropriate times, and to make documentation notations on a special form that will go in the medical record, would score a "3." It does not really alter deep, fundamental paradigms (the meds are still under the control of the nurse who is still involved in the process, documentation is still required on paper forms, etc.) but it is a clever twist on the usual process. While it picks up on the concept of "customer self-service," it does not quite rise to a score of "4."

Discussion of Pros and Cons

The proposed scale both incorporates the intuitive notion of mental distance, or unusualness of connection, and provides easily understood anchor points.

The scale would be helpful in rating the many ideas generated in a typical DirectedCreativity session in order to reflect on the distribution. Feeding back to the group the distribution in the middle of a session might provoke the group to higher levels of creativity, or might suggest specific tools and methods that could be used to fill in the gaps. For example, if there are few "4" ideas, we might try randomly suggesting other industries or using the mental benchmarking tool.

We would not want to become overly fixated on the scores of individual ideas or the distribution for a group of ideas. In the end, all that really matters is that we get at least a few ideas that are useful in addressing the issue and that are as innovative as we need them to be. A group that generates 19 "1" and "2" ideas, but one "5" idea that they eventually implement would probably be judged as more innovative than a group that generated 5 ideas each in categories "1" - "4," but selecting a "2" to implement. This rating scale is just one component of an overall approach to increasing the innovativeness of an organization.

It might be useful to allow 0.5 increments in the scale, but trying to score finer than that is probably stretching the concept too much.

The rating scale does depend somewhat on the knowledge of the raters; how much do they know about what is common in their own industry and others? The rating might also differ by national setting; that is, a concept might be rather common in British industry but not so in the US, or vice-versa.

There is the danger that the scoring could de-motivate partici-pants in a creative thinking session. Suppose someone genuinely has never heard of offering same-day appointments in health ser-vice (advance access) and comes up with this idea in a session by noticing that the current paradigm typically includes waiting for an appointment. For that person, the idea was creative and the mental action that they went through is commendable. To then tell that person that this idea only rates a score of "2" could be deflating (much like the "killer phrases" that are often cited as blocks to or-ganizational creativity). Care would obviously be needed in using the scale and in communicating results.

Paul Plsek's Depth of Innovation Scale (*Version 3, February 13, 2004*)

Select your top three ideas for consideration, describe it briefly and score it on a 1-6 scale by choosing the statement below that you think best describes it. Consider having others score your ideas as well. This may inform which ideas to begin prototyping.

1. **Usual Thinking.** This idea is the typical approach to the topic at hand. It is the way that most people in our industry (here, healthcare) handle it. Most similar teams, groups, departments, or organizations in our industry (healthcare) are already doing something very similar to this.

2. **Potential Better Practice Thinking.** This idea is an adaptation of ideas that are becoming somewhat common in other organizations in my industry (here, healthcare); but it is still a fairly new idea. Only one-third or fewer similar teams, groups, departments, or organizations in our industry (healthcare) are doing something like this.

3. **Clever Thinking.** This idea is a really clever twist on our existing ways of doing things; it is creative thinking on a small scale.

4. **Creative Connection Thinking.** This idea is a creative adaptation of ideas and concepts that are common outside my industry, but rarely used within my industry (here, ideas that are common outside healthcare, but not common within health care).

5. **Paradigm Busting Thinking.** This idea fundamentally challenges current mental models and paradigms in our industry (here, healthcare) in an uncommon way; it is creative thinking on a deeper scale.

6. **Original Thinking.** This idea is really a new concept and is truly amazing; no one has ever thought of anything like this before!

My IDEA:	My IDEA:
Description:	Description:
Rating:	Rating:
1 2 3 4 5 6	1 2 3 4 5 6

Paul Plsek© 2004 Paul E. Plsek and Associates, Inc. www.DirectedCreativity.com.
Reproduced with permission.

Appendix B: Six hats innovation evaluation

Instructions: Copy this sheet for as many ideas as you have prioritized and write the name/description of idea in the **green box**. Taking four minutes, write down as many **benefits, problems**, data, or information that might be needed, and **your gut feelings** about the idea. When finished, as a group, decide if this idea is worth pursuing as a prototype or rapid cycle test.

Innovative Idea:	
Benefits	Problems
Data Needed	Gut Feeling

Edward de Bono, Six Thinking Hats, Penguin, London 2000

YES ☐   NO ☐

References

1. Plsek PE. "Innovative thinking for the improvement of medical systems," *Annals of Internal Medicine*, 1999, **131**, 438–444.
2. Michalko M. *Thinkertoys*, 2nd edn, Ten Speed Press, Berkeley, CA, 2006.
3. Plsek PE. *Creativity, Innovation, and Quality*. ASQ Quality Press, Milwaukee, WI, 1997.
4. Paul Plsek, DirectedCreativity found at ***www.directedcreativity.com***.
5. Kelley T, Littman J. *The Art of Innovation*, Doubleday, New York, 2000, pp. 53–66.
6. de Bono, E. *Lateral Thinking: Creativity Step by Step*. Harper & Row, New York, 1970.
7. Altshuler G. *And Suddenly the Inventor Appeared*. Technical Innovation Center, Worcester, MA, 2004.
8. deBono E. *Six Thinking Hats*, Penguin Press, London, 2000.

CHAPTER 5
Prototyping and testing ideas

The ultimate goal in the innovation process is to produce a product or service that improves the lives of the user. Prototypes are mock-ups or models that reflect your innovative idea. They help you think more deeply about the idea and its feasibility, allow you to communicate your idea to others, and ultimately persuade potential supporters and funders to take the idea to a broader development and dissemination level.

It is virtually possible to create a prototype of anything, from a procedure to a product. Prototypes can be physical, experiential, digital, or mathematical. A prototype is the heart of innovation, and embraces the paradigm of acting before all the answers are in. The vast majority of ideas won't blossom into useful, new products or services; however, you can't know their fate until you build and test them. An exhortation heard at IDEO is to "fail often to succeed sooner." You never know whether an idea will fly until you make it real and test it in the light of day. For instance, the genomic revolution began with some simple model building of DNA structures by Watson and Crick. Having something tangible in your hands allows you to see where it could be improved; thus, prototyping is iterative, and some say never-ending.

Tool 1: physical models

Description
This is the most familiar of the prototypes. We have all built model airplanes or dollhouses. Physical prototypes or scale models are quick mock-ups using a wide variety of materials, including

Innovation in Action: A practical guide for healthcare teams, 1st edition.
By D. Scott Endsley. © 2010 Blackwell Publishing.

Styrofoam, cardboard, wood, metal, clay, Legos, or Lincoln Logs. Almost anything you have in your environment can be used to build a physical prototype. Keep in mind that the aim is a rapid yet convincing model that communicates your idea. Don't sweat the details and avoid wasting time adding frills. The goal is a physical object that communicates the basic idea (see Styrofoam robots above). It is very helpful to have individuals on your innovation team that have skills and experience with wood or metal working. Physical models can begin with simple sketches of the design or process and can evolve into tangible models from a variety of materials and degree of specificity.

MedRite – Improving Medication Administration at Kaiser Permanente Senior leadership at Kaiser Permanente recognized that medication management was a significant source of error both at Kaiser and nationally, which was in great need of innovation. In 2007, two hospitals were recruited to explore opportunities for innovation. A deep dive and brainstorming with multidisciplinary teams at both hospitals identified 11 priority ideas. These were "field tested" using a rapid testing strategy that led to a narrowing of the 11 to 3 core solutions (change of workflow to incorporate the 5 rights), no interruption wear (a sash indicating the nurse was not to be disturbed during medication rounds), and a "sacred zone" that was a no interruption space for medication preparation. These three ideas were additionally tested at both hospitals, with increasing lengths of tests focused on "how would you make it better." Based on inputs during the field test, the three components were refined. For example, the "'no interruption wear" went through a series of design modifications based on nurse feedback. When a near final prototype was ready, the full innovation was pilot tested over 3 months in the two hospitals, with collection of metrics on outcomes (medication errors, interrupts), processes, and balancing (satisfaction). These data were incorporated into the innovation change package that was disseminated throughout Kaiser Permanente regions.

Sketching

A step in the innovation process that is often overlooked is sketching. Most people work with the assumption that they cannot draw or that they are not artistic, so they should not attempt to sketch out ideas. This assumption should quickly be removed from the innovation process. Everyone can sketch at some level. The idea behind sketching is not to create a museum quality work of art or to impress anyone with your artistic skills but to simply communicate your ideas to others.

A quick 5-minute sketch or set of sketches can eliminate hours of fruitless conversations. The old adage that a picture is worth a thousand could not be more true than in the world of design. Sketching can be looked at as the language of design and can be used to convey enormous amounts of information within some very simple doodles. Simple rough sketches should not be underestimated as a tool to assist in the innovation process and should be a starting point for any innovation project. Nothing else comes close to the speed at which you can examine concepts, solve major issues, and work out changes to those concepts than using a pencil and a clean sheet of paper. Use a pencil, a ballpoint pen, a felt-tip pen, a crayon, or anything else that you feel comfortable using, but get your concepts down on paper.

There have been many world-changing, innovative concepts that started out as a smudgy sketch on a piece of paper or a cocktail napkin. (See A.G. Bell's sketch in Figure 5.1.)

Sketch your concept in many different ways. Change angles; sketch details like buttons or internal components. You should use the sketching process to truly investigate your concept. Most importantly, be honest with yourself. You should be attempting to find the weaknesses in your concept so that these weaknesses can be addressed.

Sketches can take on many forms depending on the concept.

"Napkin sketches"
Stick figures
Schematics
Flowcharts
Storyboards
Experience boards

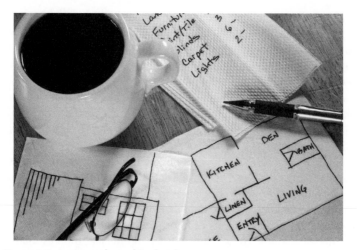

Figure 5.1 An example napkin sketch.

Sketching resources

A number of excellent guides exist to help the new innovator in learning and applying visualization techniques including sketching. These include *Rapid Viz: A New Method for the Rapid Visualization of Ideas* by Kurt Hanks and Larry Belliston. Another excellent guide is *Draw! A Visual Approach to Thinking, Learning, and Communicating* by Corinne Hanks.

Physical modeling techniques

After playing with some simple sketches you should move on to making some rudimentary representations of the physical form of your concept. These are commonly referred to as "study models," and for very good reason. This is an opportunity to examine the concept from all sides. There will be an occasional concept that has no physical form like a Web site or computer program, but even these concepts can benefit from some physical modeling of the components within the system.

Physical modeling can be a rewarding exercise and should also not be overlooked. Bringing your concept into the 3D world can bring about major revelations that might never be reached with simple sketching alone. Again, it cannot be overemphasized that this is not an artistic endeavor. You are using these physical models as another tool to investigate your concept.

Physical modeling should also be approached with an open mind and an almost childlike wonder. It is sometimes helpful to think like a 5-year-old. Anything can be used to create your study models. Several different study models should be made using different materials. Some will be more successful than others but that is the point. Even professional designers use this technique to work out details in concepts. A single trip to a local arts and crafts store such as Michael's or JoAnn's will be all you will need to get started.

Common materials and tools used to make study models are:

> Common printer paper
> Construction paper
> Bristol board
> Cardboard
> Modeling clay
> Toilet paper rolls
> Paper towel rolls
> Wooden dowels
> Foam-core board
> Beaded Styrofoam
> X-Acto knife
> Hot glue gun
> Urethane foam
> Tictacs (for buttons)
> Plywood
> Medium density fiberboard
> Wire coat hangers
> Plastic wrap
> Fun foam
> Toothpicks
> Wood glue
> Play-Doh (seriously)
> Anything!

Have fun with this stage. Go a little crazy. This is usually a fun experience and the fun of it all can lead you to observations that my have been overlooked in the "over 5-year-old" world. Remember, there is *no* wrong way to approach this phase of design.

Use

1. Define the idea for the innovation
2. Decide if a physical model would be the best way to prototype

3. Identify materials to make the prototype
4. Sketch out a rough form of prototype on paper
5. Keep it simple without frills
6. Does the prototype communicate your idea?

Tool 2: computer-aided design

Description

With the advent of high-speed computing, prototypes can be rapidly constructed within a virtual environment. Computer-aided design (CAD) software applications allow easy 2D or 3D building of a virtual object. Moreover, these applications can also create virtual environments in which your ideas could be used. These virtual reality applications allow the user to "walk around" the object, and "use" it in an electronic environment. When coupled to computer-aided manufacturing (CAM) applications and hardware, the computer design can be translated into tangible prototypes, often made in clay or plastic. Applications such as AutoCAD or TurboCAD are available for a desktop PC. It is worthwhile to get training in the use of the applications before launching into computer-aided design projects.

Although CAD and CAM processes have been around since the early 1970s, the last 10 years have brought about significant changes in the cost of these tools and the skills needed to implement them in the design process. For decades CAD/CAM has been the realm of engineers and computer programmers using large expensive computer systems and relying on specialized training. However, tools exist today that allow individuals with even a very basic understanding of engineering and a fairly average PC to implement these tools to move their designs forward.

One of the most common CAD tools used in the design world today is a PC-based program known as SolidWorks. SolidWorks can be run on just about any modern dual-core Pentium-based desktop or laptop computer, although some consideration might need to be given to memory expansion on some systems. SolidWorks allows the user to create simple 3D representations of a product or a fully manufacturable part that could be prototyped using current 3D printing techniques (see "Rapid prototyping" section).

SolidWorks is not inexpensive, with retail prices starting around $4000 but it certainly not out of the reach of the serious innovator.

Common software packages are:

SolidWorks: *www.solidworks.com*
AutoDesk Inventor: *www.autodesk.com/inventor*
Pro/Engineer: *www.proengineer.com*

Rapid prototyping

The last 5 years have seen the advent of what is referred to as rapid prototyping. This is a quick manufacturing process that can create full-sized realistic 3D components that can be used for design investigations. These parts can be produced in as little as a few hours and can be painted and finished to create realistic looking prototypes that can be used to further investigate design decisions or to communicate design intent to others.

There are several technologies that can produce these prototypes and there are hundreds of companies that can provide rapid prototyping services in just about any market.

The rapid prototyping process should not be used as the first step in the modeling process, but in the advanced stages of development rapid prototyping can be a valuable tool. Simple parts like the one at the right can be produced using rapid prototyping processes for as little as $100.

Tool 3: paper prototyping

Description

These techniques provide for creating service or product use cases over time and/or space. In many ways, these techniques extend the concept of sketching into near real world applications. Two of the most common paper prototyping techniques are storyboarding and business process mapping.

Storyboarding

This technique is commonly used in creative arts such as filmmaking and animation. It can neatly work for prototyping a service or experience, as well as use of a product innovation. Storyboards are traditionally done on paper but can also be done electronically using graphics tools such as PowerPoint.

Use
1. Obtain a 1-3 panel poster board
2. Define the "scenes" that will be displayed. These can be time based or physical space based or both
3. Sketch our actors and action for each scene
4. Post in sequence
5. Label and annotate each scene

Resources
There are a number of software tools that help a new innovator master the process of producing a storyboard such as *Storyboard Quick* (***www.powerproduction.com***). The Institute for Healthcare Improvement has developed a tool to help guide storyboard production, which can be found at ***www.ihi.org/IHI/Topics/Improvement/ ImprovementMethods/Tools/Storyboards.htm***.

Process mapping
As described in Chapter 3, the process mapping lays out the sequence or flow of materials and information through a defined process. This is useful not only to understand a current practice but also to design a new or redesigned process.

Use
1. Define the start and end points of the process that is being prototyped
2. Using the symbols in Table 5.1, construct a flow map following the designed sequence, indicating where materials and information are used or exchanged
3. Annotate at each step what the expected outcomes are anticipated
4. It is helpful if a current state process map has been produced to display the old and new processes side by side on a poster board

Resources
The American Society for Quality provides a process mapping tool that describes the approach to creating a process map which can be found at ***www.asq.org/learn-about-quality/process- analysis-tools/overview/flowchart.html***. The Institute for Healthcare Improvement also provides a useful summary guide for process mapping at ***www.ihi.org/IHI/Topics/Improvement/***

Table 5.1 Flowchart symbols

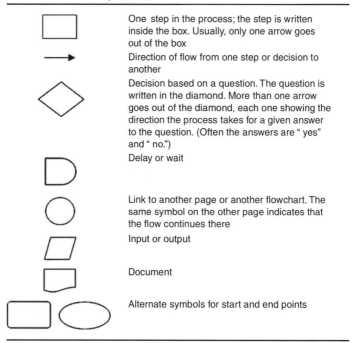

	One step in the process; the step is written inside the box. Usually, only one arrow goes out of the box
	Direction of flow from one step or decision to another
	Decision based on a question. The question is written in the diamond. More than one arrow goes out of the diamond, each one showing the direction the process takes for a given answer to the question. (Often the answers are " yes" and " no.")
	Delay or wait
	Link to another page or another flowchart. The same symbol on the other page indicates that the flow continues there
	Input or output
	Document
	Alternate symbols for start and end points

ImprovementMethods/Tools/Flowchart.htm. When process time and accuracy of each step are included in the map, you are creating a "value stream map," which is a central component to Lean Design.[1] The Lean Enterprise Institute has written a guide on value stream mapping that is extremely useful for learning to construct current and future state process maps called *Learning to See*,[2] which is available on the Lean Enterprise Institute Web site: *www.lean.org*.

Tool 4: experience prototypes

Description
These are experiential models that allow the user to experience and interact with the design idea. They can be extensions of physical prototypes or can be scenarios of service innovations. They can be set up as a museum exhibition to allow the user to move

through the scene and "use" the physical prototype or see it "used." The scenario can also be captured in short video presentations that demonstrate the user experience. Use of virtual reality applications may allow the user to virtually move through the scenario. These simulated experiences not only allow the user to see and feel the innovation but also allows the designer to examine user constraints of interaction as well as user acceptance, and redesign as needed.

Use
1. Define the innovation idea
2. Describe the scenario in which the user can experience the physical prototype or the service innovation
3. Set up the scenario with appropriate space and props
4. Provide opportunity for potential users and others to interact
5. Observe the user interactions and collect their feedback

Example
Nokia developed a prototype of an image capture and transmittal devise for children (now part of their cell phone technology). They provided these working mock-ups to children and let them carry them during their normal day. They subsequently collected information from the children on interest, use and usability, and experience of carrying an image system around with them.

Resources
The IDEO's experience with experience prototyping is well described in the paper by Buchenau and Suri available at ***http://www.ideo.com/images/uploads/thinking/publications/pdfs/FultonSuriBuchenau-Experience_PrototypingACM_8-00.pdf***.

Tool 5: mathematical models

Description
Some innovation ideas may be so small or so large as to not be easily prototyped using physical or experiential methods. For instance, a new enzyme that catalyzes intracellular cholesterol metabolism might best be modeled describing its mathematical properties. On the other end of the spectrum, a public health innovation that impacts the spread of a disease through a population is also best modeled in mathematical form.

Mathematical models can be classified in the following ways:

1. *Linear vs nonlinear*: Mathematical models are usually composed of variables, which are abstractions of factors in the described systems, and operators that act on these variables. Operators include algebraic operators, functions, and differential operators. If all the operators in a mathematical model present linearity, the resulting mathematical model is defined as linear. Otherwise, a model is considered to be nonlinear.

    The question of linearity and nonlinearity depends on context, and linear models may have nonlinear expressions in them. For example, in a statistical linear model, it is assumed that a relationship is linear in the parameters, but it may be nonlinear in the predictor variables. Similarly, a differential equation is said to be linear if it can be written with linear differential operators, but it can still have nonlinear expressions in it. In a mathematical programming model, if the objective functions and constraints are represented entirely by linear equations, then the model is regarded as a linear model. If one or more of the objective functions or constraints are represented with a nonlinear equation, then the model is known as a nonlinear model.

    Nonlinearity, even in fairly simple systems, is often associated with environments and phenomena that exhibit characteristics of complex adaptive systems, and are common in healthcare settings and biologic or physiologic phenomena. In general, nonlinear models are more difficult to mathematically model than linear ones.

2. *Deterministic vs probabilistic (stochastic)*: A deterministic model is one in which every set of variable states is uniquely determined by parameters in the model and by sets of previous states of these variables. Therefore, deterministic models perform the same way for a given set of initial conditions. Conversely, in a stochastic model, randomness is present, and variable states are not described by unique values, but rather by probability distributions. Most health systems are highly probabilistic.

3. *Static vs dynamic*: A static model does not account for the element of time, while a dynamic model does. Dynamic models typically are represented with difference equations or differential equations.

Use
1. Define the variables for analysis
2. Determine the type of mathematical model that is most applicable

3. Determine the operation(s) needed to produce the model
4. Compute the model using analysis software
5. Identify the variables and their effect level on the outcome of interest

Resources

There are a number of standard texts and monographs on mathematical modeling that can help get you started. Michael McLaughlin's *The Very Game... A Tutorial on Mathematical Modelling* is a user-friendly starter (***www.causascientia.org/math_stat/Tutorial.pdf***). There are a number of valuable software, many freeware, that are available to provide computing assistance in constructing and conducting mathematical modeling exercises. An excellent program is the free software offered by the Centers for Disease Control and Prevention called Epi-info (***www.cdc.gov/epiinfo***) that provides guidance on both data collection and analysis, from simple counts and averages to complex regression analyses. Other useful freeware tools include Dataplot (***www.itl.nist.gov/div898/software/dataplot/***) and CRAN (the R Project) at ***www.r-project.org/***. The "statistical modeling" Web site is a helpful tool for learning about different statistical testing (***tramss.data-archive.ac.uk/StatisticalModelling/index.asp***).

Tool 6: rapid cycle tests of change

Description

Before seeking funding to disseminate the innovative idea that you have prototyped (whether process or product), it is highly valuable to test whether the idea makes a difference in clinical outcome, experience of provider or patient, or administrative outcome. Rapid cycle tests of change are a part of the larger quality improvement set of strategies with which many healthcare organizations are familiar. In particular, it is the rapid cycle tests of change that are central to the Plan–Do–Study–Act (PDSA) improvement cycle proposed by Tom Nolan. Figure 5.2 presents the improvement model.

Use

1. Define the innovation idea
2. Plan the test (who, where, when, what, for how long)
3. Conduct the brief test

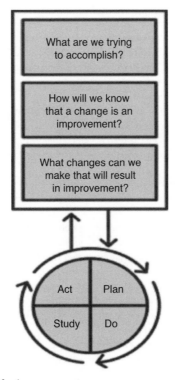

Figure 5.2 Model for improvement.

4. Measure the intended outcomes
5. Evaluate whether the innovation prototype makes a difference

The key to rapid cycle tests of change is that they are small scale and rapid. In a way, they are a variation of an experience proto-type. For instance, select to use the innovation prototype with one provider on a small handful of patients for a day or a week. Mea-sure whether the provider and/or patients detect a positive change and how easy or difficult the prototype is to use/do (Table 5.2).

Resources

There are many resources on conducting tests of change. Don Berwick, MD, the president of the Institute for Healthcare Im-provement, has summarized the rationale and methods of doing rapid cycle tests of change.[3] Tom Nolan, the designer of the PDSA

Table 5.2 Improvement tips

1. **Stay a cycle ahead.** When designing a test, imagine at the start what the subsequent test or two might be, given various possible findings in the "Study" phase of the Plan–Do–Study–Act cycle. For example, teams that are redesigning same-day admission criteria should also be planning how those criteria will be applied.

2. **Scale down the scope of tests.** Dimensions of the tests that can be scaled down include the number of patients, doctors, and others involved in the test ("Sample the next 10" instead of "Get a sample of 200"), and the location or duration of the test ("Test it in Operating Room #1 for one week").

3. **Pick willing volunteers. Work with those who want to work with you.** ("I know Dr. Jones will help us" instead of "How can we convince Dr. Smith to buy in?")

4. **Avoid the need for consensus, buy-in, or political solutions.** Save these for later stages. When possible, choose changes that do not require a long process of approval, especially during the early testing phase.

5. **Don't reinvent the wheel.** Instead, replicate changes made elsewhere. For example, instead of creating your own atrial fibrillation treatment protocol, try modifying another hospital's protocol.

6. **Pick easy changes to try.** Look for the concepts that seem most feasible and will have the greatest impact.

7. **Avoid technical slowdowns.** Don't wait for the new computer to arrive; try recording test measurements and charting trends with paper and pencil instead.

8. **Reflect on the results of every change.** After making a change, a team should ask: What did we expect to happen? What did happen? Were there unintended consequences? What was the best thing about this change? The worst? What might we do next? Too often, people avoid reflecting on failure. Remember that teams often learn very important lessons from failed tests of change.

9. **Be prepared to end the test of a change.** If the test shows that a change is not leading to improvement, the test should be stopped. Note: "Failed" tests of change are a natural part of the improvement process. If a team experiences very few failed tests of change, it is probably not pushing the boundaries of innovation very far.

model, has summarized how to conduct a PDSA including rapid cycle tests of change at *www.ihi.org/IHI/Topics/Improvement/ ImprovementMethods/HowToImprove/testingchanges.htm*.

Appendix A provides a worksheet to help you organize and manage a rapid cycle tests of change.

An innovation story continued

The elements of the new discharge were developed with support from the Greenfield Hospital discharge staff, IT staff, and a
partnership with Intel. When assembled and ready for testing, the
CCU (coronary care unit) step down volunteered to be the test site.
The CCU step down unit staff was presented the elements of the
new discharge and selected elderly patients with congestive heart
failure as the focus. Patients were recruited for a 1-month test and
informed that they were participating in an innovation project to
improve the transitions of care. Two metrics were defined for the
prototype demonstration that included (a) readmissions within
30 days and (b) patient's self-assessment of self-efficacy of home
management collected by outreach calls on a weekly basis during
the trial period. After the first month, there were 36% fewer
admissions within 30 days than during the same period of the
previous year. In addition, patients reported an overall self-efficacy
score of 7.8 out of 10.

Appendix A: worksheet for planning/conducting rapid cycle tests of change

Aim: (overall goal you wish to achieve)

Every goal will require multiple smaller tests of change

Describe your first (or next) test of change:	Person responsible	When to be done	Where to be done

Plan

List the tasks needed to set up this test of change	Person responsible	When to be done	Where to be done

Predict what will happen when the test is carried out	Measures to determine if prediction succeeds

Do   Describe what actually happened when you ran the test

Study Describe the measured results and how they compared to the predictions

Act   Describe what modifications to the plan will be made for the next cycle from what you learned

References

1. Institute for Healthcare Improvement, " Going Lean in Healthcare," found at: ***www.ihi.org/IHI/Results/WhitePapers/GoingLeaninHealthCare.htm.***
2. Rother M, Shook J. *Learning to See*, LEI, Boston, 1999.
3. Berwick DM. " Developing and Testing Changes in the Delivery of Care," *Annals of Internal Medicine*, 1998, **128** (8), 651–656.

CHAPTER 6
Creating your diffusion plan

Now that you have created a prototype and perhaps have tested it on a small scale, it is time to create a plan for spreading it within your own organization or within the marketplace (or both). Understanding the possible diffusion pathways, the factors that facilitate or constrain diffusion, and the communication/marketing strategies that might be needed is crucial for getting your innovation to market. The first step is convincing your sponsor, your organization, or potential producer/distributor that your innovation is worth investing their time and money in developing the spread programs to take the innovation beyond the prototype stage.

Diffusion of innovations

Powerful, evidence-based ideas can explode into the marketplace (e.g., use of drug-eluting stents) or take a slower route to acceptance in the medical community. For instance, a full 265 years after compelling evidence was revealed demonstrating that vitamin C-containing fruits and vegetables can prevent scurvy in sailors during long voyages, the British Royal Navy officially made vitamin C replacement standard policy.

Research on the diffusion of medical innovations has its origin in the 1950s work of James Coleman and his Columbia University team of researcher.[1] They studied the adoption of a new antibiotic, tetracycline, in four rural communities in Illinois. It was found that there were two distinct patterns of adoption—a rapid uptake of the innovation by those who were exposed to mass media messages and a slower uptake by those based on social network connections—i.e., those who knew others using tetracycline were more like to adopt themselves. More recent studies have confirmed these two pathways and have found innovations to be predominantly channeled

Innovation in Action: A practical guide for healthcare teams, 1st edition.
By D. Scott Endsley. © 2010 Blackwell Publishing.

into one of the two pathways. For instance, a recent study using the Bass model for analysis found that adoption of electronic health records in ambulatory medical practices is 20 times more impacted by influences within the social network of adopters than by factors outside the social network, such as marketing campaigns, regulatory changes, and Federal mandates.[2]

Knowledge exchange at Memorial Hospital and Health System. Memorial Hospital and Health System uses an electronic knowledge exchange that tracks and displays the innovation projects that have been completed or are ongoing across the system. A "open for picking" icon is displayed if the hospital unit welcomes visitors to come learn about their innovation. Memorial also supports an "e2 speed-dating" forum that brings together innovators from the health system with local and regional entrepreneurs to share projects.

Rogers' diffusion of innovation model

Over the past 50 years, the field of innovation diffusion has been strongly influenced by the work of Everett Rogers whose seminal work is *Diffusion of Innovations*,[3] now in its 4th edition. His study of innovations across a broad range of industries, including healthcare, suggest that the rate of innovation follows an "S"-shaped curve and that the adoption history of an innovation distinguishes different "types" of adopters at different milestones in the adoption cycle. Figure 6.1 presents the traditional S curve that is associated with

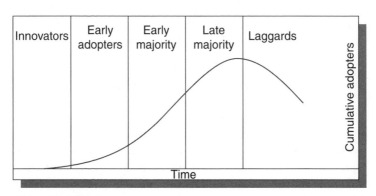

Figure 6.1 Diffusion curve.

Table 6.1 Innovator types

Type	% of total	Characteristics
Innovator	2.5	Venturesome, risk taking, contacts dispersed
Early adopter	13.5	Locally well integrated, leaders/role models
Early majority	34	Deliberate, interconnected in local system
Late majority	34	Skeptical, constrained by social norms or economic realities, low tolerance for uncertainty
Laggards	16	No leadership, rooted in past/tradition, default is status quo

Rogers' work. It should be noted that there are at least two (social network dependent and social network independent) curves that can be represented, both of which are variants on the S-shaped curve. For instance, the social network curve defined by the Bass model[4] has a slow up-curve but often plateaus out at a higher adoption rate than the nonsocial network curve, which has a rapid up-curve but plateaus out at a lower adoption rate. Also important to note is that the "take-off" or tipping point of innovation diffusion (up inflection on the curve) comes at 15–20% (innovator–early adopter groups; see Table 6.1). This has implications for creating your diffusion plan.

Innovator types

Rogers further identified five types of innovation adopters: innovators, early adopters, early majority, late majority, and laggards.[3] Innovators represent 2.5% of innovation adopters, and are the most venturesome and greatest risk takers. They are usually the first adopters and often the progenitor of the innovation. Early adopters represent 13.5% of the adoption pool, and are leaders and role models who are well integrated into their networks. They jump into an innovation often before there is convincing evidence that it works. Early majority adopters represent about 34% of adopters, and are more deliberate in their adoption decision than innovators or early adopters. They often require evidence that an innovation has the potential to work before adopting. Late majority adopters represent another 34% of the adoption pool, and are characterized by low tolerance for uncertainty and high skepticism. They often voice the prohibitions of social norms or economic realities in adoption considerations. Finally, laggards are the remaining 16% who are highly constrained by the status quo, and often don't adopt innovations even after much of their network has adopted. It should be pointed out that these five types are *not* personality types but rather innovation-specific tendencies toward adoption by individuals. Thus, an individual might be an early adopter for one innovation but a laggard for another innovation.

Ten dynamics of innovation diffusion

Rogers also identified ten dynamics that facilitate or impede the diffusion of innovation.[9] These include aspects of the innovation itself, the social and environmental construct of communication and influence, and aspects of the user/adopter. These include:

- *Relative advantage*: Perceived and/or real value that the innovation provides to the user in comparison to current practice
- *Trialability:* Ability of potential users to try the innovation without commitment
- *Observability:* Degree to which potential users see others using the innovation
- *Communications channels:* Use of specific channels through which opinion leaders and early adopters can transmit their experiences, outcomes, and opinions to others in their local social networks and more distant connections
- *Homophilous groups:* How homogeneous that target groups are based on key characteristics
- *Pace of innovation/reinvention:* Degree to which the innovation is evolved during the diffusion process. All innovations are "adapted" by users to some extent—some more than others
  - *Norms, roles, social networks:* How groups are interconnected in terms of relationships
  - *Opinion leaders:* Presence and influence of individuals who are respected leaders
  - *Compatibility:* Extent to which the innovation is aligned with user's current knowledge, skills, attitudes, and beliefs
  - *Infrastructure:* Presence of existing infrastructure that supports the innovation. For example, CT scanners are dependent on computers and software infrastructure to store and display CT information

Appendix A provides some tips on how to use each of these factors in your diffusion strategy for your innovation. Appendix B provides a template for creating your own innovation diffusion plan that is modeled on the Rogers' diffusion dynamics above.

Diffusion of MedRite at Kaiser Permanente. Kaiser Permanente and its innovation consultancy compiled the results of the MedRite medication administration prototype into an innovation change package that was presented to innovation leaders at regional hospitals at a one-day kick-off meeting. This innovation change package provided the tools for implementation as well as the history of the innovation and results of the prototype test. It included not only implementation tools but also monitoring metrics to allow hospitals to track success of the translation of the innovation in their setting.

Greenhalgh diffusion of innovation model

More recently, a comprehensive systematic review of innovation diffusion factors and strategies has been completed by Trish Greenhalgh and colleagues for the British Institute for Healthcare Innovation and Improvement.[5] They have assembled a heuristic model for studying and promoting healthcare innovation diffusion (Fig. 6.2).

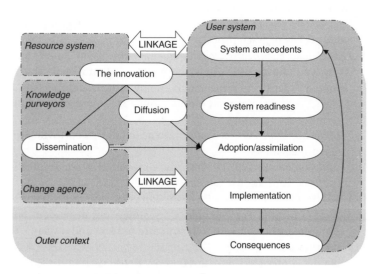

Figure 6.2 Greenhalgh diffusion model.[2]

In general, this model proposes that innovation diffusion is determined by the nature of the innovation, dissemination strategies that are employed, the attributes and readiness of the potential user system, the external environment (regulatory, financial), the linkages between the potential user system(s) and the innovators as well as external resource providers.

Use of social networks

History of social network research

Beginning with the Coleman tetracycline study in the 1950s, there has been a long history of research that suggests that innovation diffusion is strongly influenced by the configuration and functional relationships within social networks. Innovations percolate through networks if the connections are aligned. This includes factors such as the strength of interpersonal ties, the directionality of the ties, and the centrality of particular individuals within a cluster. The work of Stanley Milgram, who coined the phrase "six degrees of separation" in the 1960s, suggests that social networks can be highly efficient at transmitting information. He studied how long it would take on average to pass a letter from mid-America to an individual in Boston. On average, it had to change hands only six times before reaching Boston.

Networks in healthcare

An intriguing study from the United Kingdom[6] informs how you might think about approaching your innovation diffusion plan. In studying how medical directors and heads of nursing were connected within their professional responsibilities, it was found that heads of nursing tend to be more central within hierarchical clusters, which favors them as sources of and disseminators of information. (called "mavens" in Malcom Gladwell's book *The Tipping Point*). The medical directors were much less hierarchically linked with colleagues and tended to be embedded in highly dense clusters with high degree of connections (and less centralization of connection). In Tipping Point language, they are "connectors." These peer-to-peer linkages facilitate the rapid dissemination of innovations. This finding is supported by the Ford study that suggests it is these peer–to-peer linkages that determine the speed of adoption of electronic information technologies in the United States.

How do networks help innovation diffusion?

So how do social network configurations and functions produce different patterns of innovation diffusion, and what are their implications for formulating a diffusion plan? It has been suggested that there are three possible mechanisms.[7] First, linkages between individuals affiliated with different clusters (weak ties) might serve to pollinate each cluster with innovations. One benefit, for example, of state medical society meetings is to allow networking of acquaintances from across the state, sharing their experiences, and possibly new ideas. Second, innovations introduced by peripheral members of a densely linked cluster (e.g., medical directors) might percolate efficiently through the cluster. Finally, innovations introduced by highly linked individuals (high degrees of centrality like the heads of nursing) will effectively diffuse to the connections of this highly connected (and often highly respected) individual. This network configuration is known as a "scale-free" network in which the vast majority of individuals are connected to just a few central people. Google uses this network principle to run its Internet search engine, producing search results in nanoseconds by starting the search with the most connected sites. A classic case of this network method is the opinion leader research on new caesarian section guidelines promoted by the Canadian Society of Obstetrics and Gynecology. The results of this study suggest that opinion leaders/physician champions were the most effective means by which to change practice. Interestingly, the opinion leader doesn't need to be an early adopter himself or herself, but simply a respected individual who is knowledgeable and believable in their innovation promotion.

Hot versus simmering. Kaiser Permanente found that some innovations were "hot," meaning there was a great push to get them into implementation even before pilot testing was complete whereas others were "simmering" where there wasn't a push for implementation which allowed extended pilot testing and data collection before dissemination.

Viral/buzz marketing

The effect of social networks on spread of new ideas, behaviors, and practices has been employed by marketing companies. The marketing world understands that word of mouth or viral marketing can spread a new product like a wildfire.[8] It builds on the second network dynamic above—introduction into highly clustered networks through peripheral individuals—and relies on peer-to-peer spread. It is grounded in the human predilection for telling stories. Viral marketing starts with something to talk about (a great story). Start with creating your story—something that is taboo, unusual, outrageous, hilarious, or secret—and introduce it through trained "people on the street." The story can be augmented through demonstration of the product or service. For example, the video game industry often gives away their new games to individuals with instruction to play it in public.

In summary, social network-based strategies for innovation diffusion might encompass:

- taking advantage of individuals who are well connected outside their normal social network to promote the innovation—identify the connectors
- introducing your innovation into the periphery of networks at multiple points (i.e., viral marketing described above)
- taking advantage of opinion leaders in social networks to promote your innovation—identify the mavens

Creating your diffusion plan

Understanding the key factors that influence the diffusion of innovation is helpful to create a diffusion plan as part of your larger business plan. This outlines the characteristics of your innovation that influence diffusion, and elucidates a variety of strategies that might be used to spread your innovation throughout your organization and within the larger healthcare marketplace.

Appendix B provides a diffusion plan form that helps you formulate the elements of a diffusion plan that incorporates both social network and nonsocial network strategies. It asks you to set the foundations for your plan through specifying:

- key characteristics of your innovation
- key characteristics of your target audience

Innovation characteristics

Innovation characteristics include the relative advantage of your innovation over existing products or services, the complexity/ease of use of the innovation, how adaptable it is by users, how compatible the innovation is with respect to current work processes, technologies and interpersonal interactions, and dependence of the innovation on existing technologies or work processes. Recognizing that you may not have data to evaluate your innovation on these variables, record your best estimate. Consider using these parameters to monitor your innovation spread and adjusting your diffusion strategies based on information that arises from the spread process.

Target audience characteristics

Potential user characteristics include their demographics (age, sex, position in the healthcare system), the homogeneity/homophily of this group, how they are linked both within themselves and to other clusters of people within the organization, healthcare system or medical community, and other defining characteristics that might define how "ready" they are for adopting your innovation. As with the characteristics of your innovation, this information may not be fully known and may need to be monitored during the diffusion stage. For instance, you may discover that your innovation is actually being used by a different age group or role within the healthcare system.

Select your diffusion strategies

Consider how you will approach spreading your innovation both within your organization and outside your organization within the larger medical marketplace. How will you solicit approval, support, funding to proceed? Who will be the opinion leaders/influentials you might use to spread the innovation? How might you use viral marketing to get your innovation used? Are there nonsocial network strategies that you might employ, such as advertising, mass media campaigns, opportunities to align/change regulatory policy? How will you ensure that potential users of your innovation have a chance to try it out and/or observe others using it? Appendix A provides some tips on things to consider.

Tools for communicating your innovation

Critical to any innovation diffusion strategy is the ability to effectively inform and persuade the target audiences you have defined in your diffusion plan. Mass media marketing may be an element in your communication strategy, which is beyond the scope of this action guide. Messages directed at internal leadership and potential users as well as the medical community networks outside your organization also play a critical role in how successfully your innovation is spread. Below are three "tools" for communication that you might find helpful.

Tool 1: storyboard

Description

A storyboard is a graphical presentation that enables the innovator to describe the innovation, its uses, and its benefits (Fig. 6.3). When coupled with the actual physical prototype, it can be a compelling way to communicate the development and future of your innovation. There are numerous formats for creating a storyboard. Some key elements to include are:
- the name of the innovation
- the innovation team (names, photos)

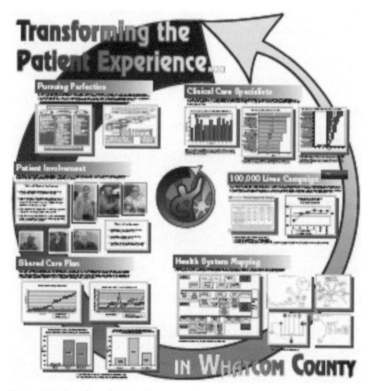

Figure 6.3 Storyboard example.

- innovation sponsors
- statement of the innovation challenge
- assessment strategies used and results
- description of the innovation
- projected future of the innovation

Great storyboards are brief, highly graphical, and a mix of images, data, and text, and they focus on how the innovation meets the innovation challenge. They also allow interaction with the innovation, if possible, through a physical or experience prototype.

Use

1 Draw out the proposed format of the storyboard
2 Obtain a storyboard (from any office supply store)
3 Assemble the defined elements (images, graphs, text boxes)
4 On a flat surface, lay the storyboard down and place elements where you would want them to go
5 If the team is in agreement, proceed with affixing these elements to the storyboard
6 Prepare a presentation that highlights the elements on the storyboard
7 Conduct the presentation to the sponsor, funder, or producer

Resources

The Institute for Healthcare Improvement has developed a tool to help teams produce a storyboard representing the process and outcomes of improvement efforts at *www.ihi.org/IHI/Topics/ Improvement/ImprovementMethods/Tools/Storyboards.htm.*

Tool 2: videography

Description

Larger innovations may not be compressible onto a storyboard or service/process innovations; a dramatic way of presenting the new design is through a video presentation. This video is simple yet compelling as it lays out the design process and the new service, and demonstrates it (such as an experience prototype).

Use

1 Write out the script and flow of the video presentation
2 Rehearse the presentation
3 When comfortable with presentation, video it

4 Do appropriate editing; keep it short—5–8 minutes
5 Present it to the target individuals/audience

Tool 3: viral/buzz marketing

Description

Humans love a good story, and love telling stories. How can you weave a story that informs and convinces others in social networks to try your innovation? The advantage of viral messages is that your message is being provided face to face without other media distractions, and through nonthreatening, noninvasive human interaction. It is about starting a conversation that at some point involves your innovation.

Use

1 Craft a story (see the "six buttons of buzz" in Table 6.2)
2 Identify individuals within the networks you'd like to influence
3 Provide them the story (you may pay them as viral marketers)
4 Allow them to embellish and adapt the story based on their audiences
5 Update the story(s) as needed

Resources

The Word of Mouth Marketing Association (yes, there is a buzz trade association) has useful links and resources at *http://www.womma.org/*. Mark Hughes, one of the gurus of viral marketing, has is own Web site (and book that he promotes) at www.buzzmarketing.com. There are numerous books on viral/buzz marketing. My favorite is *The Anatomy of Buzz* by Emanuel Rosen.[8]

Table 6.2 Six buttons of buzz

1.	The taboo (sex, lies, bathroom humor)
2.	The unusual
3.	The outrageous
4.	The hilarious
5.	The remarkable
6.	Secrets

*Source: **www.buzzmarketing.com**.*

Creating your story

The best ways of diffusing your innovation as described above is through developing and using connections between people in a social network. But to do this, you need to catch and hold their attention. This can be done through development of a good story about your innovative service or product that portrays meaning and relevance to the potential users in the social network. A good story also allows your potential user to remember your service or product, and retell the story to others in their own way.

Start developing your storyline during your deep dive as you listen and observe the needs, values, preferences, and stories of people. What would you want these networks of people to say about your service or product? What needs does your service or product improve, and how does it make their lives better? As you design your storyboard or other display, it is not just information that you are conveying but, more importantly, a story about your product or service. Some things to consider in formulating your marketing story are:

- What is your strong, central theme? Can you express it in one line like a newspaper headline?
- What things do the main character(s) share with your audience?
- What kind of setting/environment does your story take place?
- What kind of "zing" can you insert (see six buttons of buzz in Table 6.2)?

Appendix C provides a guide for putting your story together for your diffusion plan.

Measuring the reach and impact of the innovation

As you launch into your dissemination/distribution efforts based on your diffusion plan, measuring the acceptance, use, and impact of your innovation is crucial. Consider selecting a small, "balanced scorecard" that provides metrics on use, clinical impact, financial impact, and user satisfaction, which is a good way to start.[9] Table 6.3 presents a model scorecard that provides a template for your efforts to establish metrics that track whether your innovation makes a difference. These metrics can be adapted as you move from internal dissemination to external distribution.

Table 6.3 Innovation scorecard

Innovation use	• Proportion of intended audience ever using innovation
	• Proportion of intended audience using innovation on daily basis
	• Proportion of intended audience correctly using innovation
Clinical impact	• % change in tended clinical outcome (e.g., lower A1C rate)
	• % change in service utilization (e.g., ED visits)
	• % change in knowledge of provider and/or patients
Financial impact	• % and absolute change in cost per unit service
	• % change in organizational revenues
User satisfaction	• % change in user experience score

Key considerations in assembling your scorecard will be the following:
• Data sources: use already existing sources, if possible
• Frequency of measurement
• Who will be responsible for measurement
• How will you present and use the measurement

Consider putting together a report sheet that can be distributed to the innovation team as well as the executive team in your organization. Use it for internal discussion in the team to evaluate possible redesigns of your innovation. The scorecard will also give you a good sense of when the innovation might be ready to take to a wider audience or market. For example, an innovation that is used appropriately and fits into common work patterns, produces significant changes in disease conditions and service utilization, saves the organization money or provides an appreciable revenue stream, and is well accepted by users is "market ready."

Don't spend a lot of time inventing metrics to use for your scorecard. There are a number of national resources that provide libraries of validated measures that can be adapted for your innovation and for your organization and setting. These include:

National Quality Measure Clearinghouse: This site maintained by the Agency for Healthcare Research and Quality (AHRQ) is the largest compendium of measures in a searchable format. The Web site is: ***www.qualitymeasures.ahrq.gov.***

AMA Physician Consortium for Performance Improvement: AMA is the largest measure producer for healthcare and produces a wide array of measures (213 measures in 31 topic areas) used by Centers for Medicare and Medicaid Services (CMS) and others. Their measures can be found at ***www.ama-assn.org/ama/pub/category/4837.html.***

CMS Physician Quality Reporting Initiative (PQRI): The CMS has developed a performance measurement program that includes 119 measures. The full list of 2008 proposed measures can be found at www.cms.hhs.gov/PQRI/downloads/2008PQRIQuality MeasureSpecs123107.pdf. CMS has also produced a Web-based library of measures called the Quality Measurement Management Information System (QMIS), which contains searchable libraries of measures used not only by CMS but by other federal programs as well. It can be found at ***www.qualitynet.org/qmis/.***

Appendix D provides a template for starting your innovation dissemination scorecard.

An innovation story continued

Buoyed by the enthusiasm from both the CCU step down unit staff and the patients participating in the prototype demonstration phase, the innovation team produced a short, 5-minute video showing the new discharge as well as a storyboard. The team presented the results to the CEO and hospital board. Most impressive for the board was the presentation of the dollars saved by preventing readmissions. By unanimous vote, the board agreed to direct the CEO to fund similar discharge programs in three additional units and to continue support of the program on the CCU step down unit.

The innovation team coleaders captured the new discharge program into an easy-to-use, step-by-step innovation package, including the process by which it was designed and the results achieved in the prototype experience. They also presented the results of this innovation experiment in their local and state physician and nursing societies, and wrote a joint paper that was published in the *Joint Commission Journal on Quality and Patient Safety*. Over the ensuing months, they received increasing numbers of requests from other health systems and hospitals for their innovation package. After 6 months, they decided to charge a small fee for the innovation package, and then decided that there was a business opportunity to provide consulting services to other regional health systems interested in improving their discharge process. They proposed to the CEO who approved the formation of a part-time Greenfield Innovation Consultancy with revenue sharing between the health system and the consultancy in order to enable further development of innovation programs.

Appendix A: tips for healthcare innovation diffusion

(*used with permission*)

Adapted from Cain and Mittman (2002)[10]

Relative Advantage
- Understand the end user of the innovation
- Recognize the impact of significant behavior change
- Consider the business case for adoption of innovation

Triability
- Look for opportunities to carve out some part of a system that is "trialable"
- When designing a new technology or process system, consider which components/steps could be tried out without committing to full innovation

Observability
- Make the invisible visible with viral marketing

Communication channels
- To *inform* people about an innovation, select mass media and "cosmopolite" sources. To *persuade* people to adopt the innovation, closer links, and interpersonal channels are more effective
- To communicate more complex messages, select interpersonal communications channels
- In order to select the right communication channels, select the right target audience
- Identify people who are "connectors"

Homophilous groups
- To use homophily as an innovation promoter, understand the degree of homophily in the target group
- Look for homophilous groups beyond physicians
- Put the right individual in front of your target audience

Pace of innovation
- Put in place active listening posts
- Monitor healthcare innovations very carefully for instances of potentially dangerous misuses

- Look for workarounds that users employ to make an innovation work
- Do not be offended by reinvention

Norms, roles, and social networks
- Pay explicit attention to the physician and virtual networks of the groups you wish to reach
- Be aware of opportunities to leverage existing or to create new social networks

Opinion leaders
- Do not mistake early adopters for opinion leaders
- Work hard to identify the relevant opinion leaders
- Be on the lookout for 'mavens'

Compatibility
- Understand current behaviors and values
- Innovations that reduce hassles are more likely to be successful
- Mimic things from other parts of life

Infrastructure
- Look for opportunities to plug and play
- Understand current and future regulatory constraints and competing patent protections
- Look for leapfrogging opportunities, especially in technology

Appendix B

Innovation Diffusion Plan

Submitted By: _____

Innovation Description:

Label:

Description:

Foundation Setting

A. My Innovation (rate your innovation on these scales)

    1. Relative advantage over existing product/service

None	Little	Some	Good Advantage	Great Advantage

    Relative advantages are:

☐ Cheaper   ☐ Generates more revenue   ☐ More reliable

☐ More accurate   ☐ Easier to Use/Perform   ☐ Safer   ☐ Faster

☐ Fewer dependencies on people/technologies

    2. Complexity of Use

Requires great skill	Fair amt of additional skill required	Some additional skill required	Small additional skill required	No additional skill required

3. Adaptability of innovation by users

Not adaptable	Slightly adaptable	Moderately adaptable	Reasonably adaptable	Easily adaptable

4. Compatibility of innovation with user workflow, technologies, social patterns

Not at all compatible	Slightly compatible	Moderately compatible	Reasonably compatible	Highly compatible

5. Depends on an existing process or technology

Highly dependant	Fairly dependent	Somewhat dependent	Slightly dependent	Not at all dependant

B. My Target Audience (tick all that apply)

    1. Demographics

☐ Males   ☐ Females

☐ 1-12yrs ☐ 13-18 yrs ☐ 18-45 yrs ☐ 46-65 yrs ☐ 65+

☐ Pt families ☐ Patients ☐ Nurses ☐ Physicians ☐ Managers

☐ Administrative staff   ☐ C-Level leaders (eg CEO)

    2.   How similar/homogenous is my target audience?

Highly Different	Fairly Different	Somewhat Different	Fairly Similar	Highly Homogenous

3. How are my target audiences linked?
   ☐ highly centralized*   ☐ densely clustered**
        ☐ Ties outside of cluster***

4. What are the main characteristics of my target
   audience?

My Diffusion Strategies
A. Inside My Own Organization

☐ **CEO presentation**   ☐ **Board presentation**
☐ **Opinion leaders (who-   )**
☐ **Viral spread (describe how -   )**
☐ **Non-network strategies (describe-   )**
☐ **Opportunities for trial/observation of innovation**
(describe-   )

B. Outside of My Organization
☐ **Opinion leaders (who-   )**
☐ **Viral spread (describe how -   )**
☐ **Non-network strategies (describe-   )**
☐ **Opportunities for trial/observation of innovation**
(describe-   )

C. My Story (use humor, unusual,
   outrageous, taboo story constructs)

My Diffusion Plan Sumary
Based on the selected strategies above, my plan for spreading
my innovation will be:

Appendix C
My Diffusion Story

Title of My Story:

_____

Audience for Story: *Check all that apply*

☐ Organization's Leaders   ☐ Potential funders/investor
☐ Potential users/purchasers

> **Scene for Story:**

> **Actors:**
> ☐
> ☐

> **Theme(s)**
> ☐
> ☐

Key Events of Story and How They Relate to Theme(s):

Event	How Relates to Theme

Storyline
For the events and actors in the scene identified, how does the story unfold? Indicate sequence of events and relationship of actors, and how theme is reinforced.

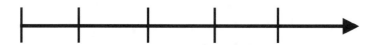

Appendix D
My Diffusion Scorecard

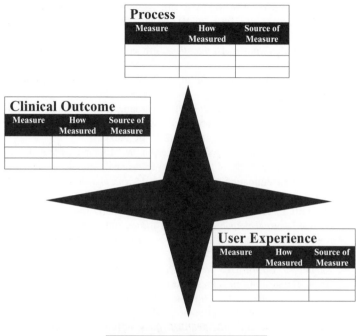

References

1. Coleman JS, Menzel H, Katz E. "The diffusion of an innovation among physicians," *Sociometry*, 1957, **20**, 253–270.
2. Ford EW, Menachemi N, Phillips MT. "Predicting the adoption of electronic health records by physicians: when will healthcare be paperless?" *Journal of the American Medical Informatics Association*, 2006, **13**, 106–112.
3. Rogers EM. *Diffusion of Innovations*, 4th edn, Free Press, New York, 1995.
4. Bass Model Research Institute available at: ***http://www.bassmodel institute.org/***
5. Greenhalgh T, Robert G, Bate P, Macfarlane F, Kyriakidou O. *Diffusion of Innovations in Health Services Organizations: A Systematic Literature Review*, Blackwell Publishing, Malden, MA, 2005.
6. West E, Barron DN, Dowsett J, Newton JN. "Hierarchies and cliques in the social networks of healthcare professionals: implications for the design of dissemination strategies," *Social Science and Medicine*, 1999, **48**, 633–646.
7. McGrath C, Krackhardt D. "Network conditions for organizational change," *Journal of Applied Behavioral Science*, 2003, **39**(3), 324–336.
8. Rosen E. *The Anatomy of Buzz: How to Create Word of Mouth Marketing*, Doubleday, New York, 2000.
9. Kaplan RS, Norton DP. *The Balanced Scorecard: Translating Strategy into Action*, Harvard Business Press, Boston, 1996.
10. Cain M, Mittman R. "Diffusion of innovation in healthcare," California HealthCare Foundation Whitepaper, May 2002, found at: ***www.chcf.org/documents/ihealth/DiffusionofInnovation.pdf***.

Appendix

Useful Web sites

IDEO: www.ideo.com

DirectedCreativity: www.directedcreativity.org

NHS Institute for Innovation and Improvement: http://www.institute.nhs.uk/

Innovation Tools: www.innovationtools.com

FutureThink: http://www.getfuturethink.com/

Agency for Healthcare Research and Quality Healthcare Innovation Exchange: http://www.innovations.ahrq.gov/

Innovation Learning Network: http://iln-public.pbwiki.com/2006%20ILN%20Learnings

Institute for the Future: http://www.iftf.org/

Clinical Microsystems: http://www.clinicalmicrosystem.org/

Institute for Healthcare Improvement: www.ihi.org

Lean Enterprise Institute: http://www.lean.org/

Global Business Network: www.gbn.com (scenario planning tools)

Innocentive: http://www.innocentive.com/

Second Life: www.secondlife.com

Center for Health Design: www.healthdesign.org

Articles

Bate P, Robert G. "Experience-based Design: From Designing the System Around the Patient to Co-Designing Services with the Patient," *Quality and Safety in Healthcare*, 2006, **15,** 307–310.

Berwick DM. "Disseminating Innovations in Healthcare," *JAMA*, 2003, **289**(15), 1969–1975.

Bradley EH, Webster TR, Baker D, et al. "Translating Research into Practice: Speeding Adoption of Innovative Healthcare Programs," 2004, found at: www.cmwf.org.

Brown T. "Strategy by Design," *Fast Company*, 2005, June, 2–4.

Bonabeau E, Meyer C. "Swarm Intelligence: A Whole New Way to Think About Business," *Harvard Business Review*, 2001, May, 107–114.

Cain M, Mittman R. "Diffusion of Innovation in Healthcare," 2002, found at: www.chcf.org.

Commonwealth Fund "Framework for a High Performance Health System in the United States," 2006, found at: www.cwmf.org.

Drucker PF. "The Discipline of Innovation," *Harvard Business Review*, 2002, August, 2–10.

Fleuren M, Wiefferink K, Paulussen T. "Determinants of innovation within healthcare organizations," *International Journal for Quality in Healthcare*, 2004, **16**(2), 107–123.

Hagel J, Brown JS. "Creation Nets: Harnessing the Potential of Open Innovation," 2006, found at: www.johnseelybrown.com.

Hargadon A, Sutton RI. "Building an Innovation Factory," *Harvard Business Review*, 2007, Spring, 93–102.

Herzlinger RE. "Why Innovation in Healthcare Is So Hard," 2006, May, 2–10.

Herzlinger RE. "Innovating in Healthcare- Framework," *Harvard Business Review*, 2006, August, 1–54.

Larson EB. "Healthcare System Chaos Should Spur Innovation," *Annals of Internal Medicine*, 2004, **140**, 639–664.

Leonard D, Rayport JF. "Spark Innovation Through Empathic Design," *Harvard Business Review*, 1997, November–December, 103–113.

McGrath C, Krackhardt D. "Network Conditions for Organization Change," *Journal of Applied Behavioral Science*, 2003, **39**(3), 324–336.

Nussbaum B. "The Power of Design," *Business Week*, 2004, May 17.

Plsek P. "Innovative Thinking for the Improvement of Medical Systems," *Annals of Internal Medicine*, 1999, **131**(6), 438–444.

Plsek P. "Spreading Good Ideas for Better Healthcare," 2000, found at: www.vha.com.

Plsek PE "Complexity and the Adoption of Innovation in Healthcare," 2003, found at: www.nihcm.org.

Plsek PE, Greenhalgh T. "The challenge of complexity in healthcare," *BMJ*, 2001, **323**, 625–628.

Rodriquez D, Soloman D. "Leadership and Innovation in a Networked World," *Innovations*, 2007, **2**(3), 3–13.

Shannon KC, Dysinger WS. "Office of the Future," 2003, found at: www.aafp.org.

Silversin J, Kornacki MJZ. "Implementaing Change: From Ideas to Reality," *Family Practice Management*, 2003, January, 57–62.

Spear SJ "Fixing Healthcare from the Inside, Today," *Harvard Business Review*, 2005, September, 2–15.

Thomke SH. "Capturing the Real Value of Innovation Tools," *MIT Sloan Management Review*, 2006, **47**(2), 24–32.

Thomke S. "Enlightened Experimentation: The New Imperative for Innovation," *Harvard Business Review*, 2001, Feburary, 67–75.

West E, Barron DN, et al. "Hierarchies and Cliques in the Social Networks of Healthcare Professionals: Implications for the Design of Dissemination Strategies," *Social Science and Medicine*, 1999, **48**, 633–646.

Wejnert B. "Integrating Models of Diffusion of Innovations: A Conceptual Framework," *Annual Review of Sociology*, 2002, **28**, 297–326.

Books

Altshuller G. *And Suddenly the Inventor Appeared: TRIZ, the Theory of Inventive Problem Solving*, Technical Innovation Center, Worcester, MA, 1994.

Amabile TM. *Creativity in Context*, Westview Press, Boulder, CO, 1996.

Burns LR (ed). *The Business of Healthcare Innovation*, Cambridge University Press, Cambridge UK, 2005.

Buzan T. *The Mind Map Book*, Plume Books, New York, 1996.

Chesbrough H. *Open Business Models*, Harvard Business Press, Boston, 2006.

Christensen, Clayton M. *The Innovator's Dilemma*. Harvard Business School Press, Boston, 1997.

Christensen, Clayton M, Raynor, ME. *The Innovator's Solution*, Harvard Business School Press, Boston, 2003.

Claxton G. *Hare Brain, Tortoise Mind*, Ecco Press, London, 1997.

Csikszentmihalyi M. *Creativity: Flow and the Psychology of Discovery and Invention*, Harper Collins, New York, 2001.

Csikszentmihalyi M. *Good Business*, Penguin, New York, 2003.

Davis K. *Getting Into Your Customers Head, Crown Business*, 1996.

De Bono E. *Lateral Thinking: Creativity Step by Step*, Harper and Row, New York, 1970.

De Bono E. *Six Thinking Hats*, Little Brown & Co., New York, 1985.

Forbes P. *The Geckos Foot*, WW Norton & Company, New York, 2005.

Goldsmith J. *Digital Medicine*, Health Administration Press, Chicago, 2003.

Gladwell, M. *The Tipping Point*, Little, Brown & Co., New York, 2000.

Greenhalgh T, Robert G, Bate P, Macfarlane F, Kyriakidou O. *Diffusion of Innovations in Health Service Organizations*, BMJ Books/Blackwell Publishing, London, 2005.

Harvard Business Review on Innovation. Harvard Business Press, Boston, 2001.

Institute of Medicine. *To Err is Human*, National Academy Press, Washington, DC, 2000.

Institute of Medicine. *Crossing the Quality Chasm*, Academy Press, Washington, DC, 2001.

Institute for the Future. *Health and Healthcare, 2010*, Jossey-Bass, San Francisco, 2003.

Johansson F. *The Medici Effect: What Elephants and Epidemics Can Teach Us About Innovation*, Harvard Business School Press, Boston, 2006.

Kelley T. *The Ten Faces of Innovation*, Doubleday, New York, 2005.

Kelley T. *The Art of Innovation, Doubleday*, New York, 2001.

Langley GJ, Nolan KM, Nolan TW, Norman CL, Provost LP. *The Improvement Guide*, Jossey-Bass, San Francisco, 1996.

Laurel B (ed). *Design Research: Methods and Perspectives*, MIT Press, Cambridge, MA, 2003.

Moggridge B. *Designing Interactions*, MIT Press, Cambridge, MA, 2007.

Myerson J. IDEO: Masters of Innovation, Laurence King Publishing, London, 2004.

Michalko M. *Cracking Creativity*, Ten Speed Press, Berkeley, 2001.

Michalko M. *Thinkertoys*, Ten Speed Press, Berkeley, 2006.

NHS. *Thinking Differently Guide*, found at: www.institute.nhs.uk /building_capability/new_model_for_transforming_the_nhs/thinking_ differently_guide.html.

Nalebuff B, Ayres I. *Why Not? How to Use Everday Ingenuity to Solve Problems Big and Small*, Harvard Business School Press, Boston, 2003.

Norman DA. *The Design of Future Things*, Basic Books, New York, 2007.

Norman DA. *The Design of Everydayt Things*, Basic Books, New York, 1988.

Pink DH. *A Whole New Mind*, Riverhead Books, New York, 2005.

Plsek P. *Creativity, Innovation and Quality*, Quality Press, Milwaukee, WI, 1997.

Porter ME, Teisberg EO. *Redefining Healthcare*, Harvard Business School Press, Boston, 2006.

Rogers EM. *Diffusion of Innovations*, Free Press, New York, 1995.

Rosen E. *The Anatomy of Buzz*, Doubleday, New York, 2000.

Silverman G. *The Secrets of Word-of-Mouth Marketing*, American Management Association, New York, 2001.

Utterback JM. *Mastering the Dynamics of Innovation*, Harvard Business Press, Boston, 1996.

Utterback J, Vedin BA, Alvarez E, Ekman S, Sanderson SW, Tether B, Verganti R. *Design-Inspired Innovation*, World Scientific, London, 2006.

Von Hippel E. *The Sources of Innovation*, Oxford University Press, Oxford, 1988.

Von Hippel E. *Democratizing Innovation*, MIT Press, Cambridge, MA, 2005.

Weick KE. *Sensemaking in Organizations*, Sage, London, 1995.

Weick KE, Sutcliffe KM. *Managing the Unexpected*, Jossey-Bass, San Francisco, 2001.

Zimmerman B, Lindberg C, Plsek P. *Edgeware: Insights from Complexity Science for Healthcare Leaders*, VHA Inc, Irving, TX, 2001.

Index

Note: Italicized page numbers refer to tables and figures